Computational
Genetic Screening

Computational Genetic Screening

Ralph Phillip

Editor

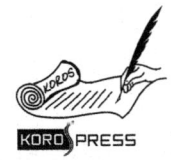

KOROS PRESS LIMITED

London, UK

Computational Genetic Screening

© 2012

Printed in 2017 for Sale in the Indian Subcontinent

Published by
Koros Press Limited
3 The Pines, Rubery B45 9FF, Rednal,
Birmingham, United Kingdom

Tel.: +44-7826-930152
Email: info@korospress.com
www.korospress.com

ISBN: 978-1-78163-197-3

Editor: Ralph Phillip

Printed in UK

British Library Cataloguing in Publication Data
A CIP record for this book is available from the British Library

10 9 8 7 6 5 4 3 2 1

Exclusively distributed by CBS Publishers & Distributors Pvt. Ltd.
Sales & Distribution Rights only for India, Pakistan, Bangladesh, Sri Lanka, Nepal and Bhutan.This book is not to be sold outside these territories.

Contents

Preface

In bioinformatics, a sequence alignment is a way of arranging the sequences of DNA, RNA, or protein to identify regions of similarity that may be a consequence of functional, structural, or evolutionary relationships between the sequences. Aligned sequences of nucleotide or amino acid residues are typically represented as rows within a matrix. Gaps are inserted between the residues so that identical or similar characters are aligned in successive columns. A sequence alignment, produced by ClustalW, of two human zinc finger proteins, identified on the left by GenBank accession number. Computational approaches to sequence alignment generally fall into two categories: *global alignments* and *local alignments*. Calculating a global alignment is a form of global optimization that "forces" the alignment to span the entire length of all query sequences. By contrast, local alignments identify regions of similarity within long sequences that are often widely divergent overall. Local alignments are often preferable, but can be more difficult to calculate because of the additional challenge of identifying the regions of similarity. A variety of computational algorithms have been applied to the sequence alignment problem, including slow but formally optimizing methods like dynamic programming, and efficient, but not as thorough heuristic algorithms or probabilistic methods designed for large-scale database search.

Alignments are commonly represented both graphically and in text format. In almost all sequence alignment representations, sequences are written in rows arranged so that aligned residues appear in successive columns. In text formats, aligned columns containing identical or similar characters are indicated with a system of conservation symbols. As in the image above, an asterisk or pipe symbol is used to show identity between two columns; other less common symbols include a colon for conservative substitutions and a period for semiconservative substitutions. Many sequence visualization programs also use colour to display information about the properties of the individual sequence elements; in DNA and RNA sequences, this equates to assigning each nucleotide its own colour.

In protein alignments, such as the one in the image above, colour is often used to indicate amino acid properties to aid in judging the conservation of a given amino acid substitution. For multiple sequences the last row in each column is often the consensus sequence determined by the alignment; the consensus sequence is also often represented in graphical format with a sequence logo in which the size of each nucleotide or amino acid letter corresponds to its degree of conservation. Sequence alignments can be stored in a wide variety of text-based file formats, many of which were originally developed in conjunction with a specific alignment program or implementation. Most web-based tools allow a limited number of input and output formats, such as FASTA format and GenBank format and the output is not easily editable. Several conversion programs are available, READSEQ or EMBOSS having a graphical interfaces or command line interfaces, while several programming packages like BioPerl, BioRuby provide functions to do this.

This book is a comprehensive and analytical study of Molecular Genetics which covers, nearly, all important aspects of DNA and molecular testing.

—*Editor*

Chapter 1

Visualising Human Chromosomes

Human Genome

The human genome is the genome of *Homo sapiens*, which is stored on 23 chromosome pairs. 22 of these are autosomal chromosome pairs, while the remaining pair is sex-determining. The haploid human genome occupies a total of just over 3 billion DNA base pairs. The Human Genome Project (HGP) produced a reference sequence of the euchromatic human genome, which is used worldwide in biomedical sciences.

The haploid human genome contains ca. 23,000 protein-coding genes, far fewer than had been expected before its sequencing. In fact, only about 1.5% of the genome codes for proteins, while the rest consists of non-coding RNA genes, regulatory sequences, introns, and noncoding DNA (once known as "junk DNA").

Features

Genes

There are estimated to be between 20,000 and 25,000 human protein-coding genes. The estimate of the number of human genes has been repeatedly revised down as genome sequence quality and gene finding methods have improved. Earlier predictions estimated that human cells have as much as 200,000 genes.

Surprisingly, the number of human genes seems to be less than a factor of two greater than that of many much simpler organisms, such as the roundworm and the fruit fly. However, human cells make extensive use of alternative splicing to produce several different proteins from a single gene, and the human proteome is thought to be much larger than those of the aforementioned organisms. Besides, most human genes have multiple exons, and human introns are frequently much longer than the flanking exons.

Human genes are distributed unevenly across the chromosomes. Each chromosome contains various gene-rich and gene-poor regions, which seem to be correlated with chromosome bands and GC-content.

The significance of these nonrandom patterns of gene density is not well understood. In addition to protein coding genes, the human genome contains thousands of RNA genes, including tRNA, ribosomal RNA, microRNA, and other non-coding RNA genes.

Regulatory Sequences

The human genome has many different regulatory sequences which are crucial to controlling gene expression. These are typically short sequences that appear near or within genes. A systematic understanding of these regulatory sequences and how they together act as a gene regulatory network is only beginning to emerge from computational, high-throughput expression and comparative genomics studies.

Some types of non-coding DNA are genetic "switches" that do not encode proteins, but do regulate when and where genes are expressed.

Identification of regulatory sequences relies in part on evolutionary conservation. The evolutionary branch between the primates and mouse, for example, occurred 70–90 million years ago. So computer comparisons of gene sequences that identify conserved non-coding sequences will be an indication of their importance in duties such as gene regulation.

Another comparative genomic approach to locating regulatory sequences in humans is the gene sequencing of the puffer fish. These vertebrates have essentially the same genes and regulatory gene sequences as humans, but with only one-eighth the noncoding DNA. The compact DNA sequence of the puffer fish makes it much easier to locate the regulatory genes.

Other DNA

Protein-coding sequences (specifically, coding exons) comprise less than 1.5% of the human genome. Aside from genes and known regulatory sequences, the human genome contains vast regions of DNA the function of which, if any, remains unknown.

These regions in fact comprise the vast majority, by some estimates 97%, of the human genome size.

Repeat Elements

- Tandem repeats;
  - — Satellite DNA
  - — Minisatellite
  - — Microsatellite.
- Interspersed repeats;
  - — SINEs
  - — LINEs.

Transposons

- Retrotransposons;
  - — [[Retrotransposon#LTR retrotransposons | LTR]]
    - – Ty1-copia
    - – Ty3-gypsy.
  - — Non-LTR
    - – SINEs
    - – LINEs
- DNA Transposons.

Noncoding DNA

There is also a large amount of sequence that does not fall under any known classification. Much of this sequence may be an evolutionary artifact that serves no present-day purpose, and these regions are collectively referred to as noncoding DNA. These regions were once referred to as "junk" DNA; however, there are a variety of emerging indications that many sequences within are likely to function in ways that are not fully understood.

Recent experiments using microarrays have revealed that a substantial fraction of non-genic DNA is in fact transcribed into RNA, which leads to the possibility that the resulting transcripts may have some unknown function. Also, the evolutionary conservation across the mammalian genomes of much more sequence than can be explained by protein-coding regions indicates that many, and perhaps most, functional elements in the genome remain unknown.

The investigation of the vast quantity of sequence information in the human genome whose function remains unknown is currently a major avenue of scientific inquiry. Meanwhile, considering the global genome DNA information as a whole could provide new ways to understand a possible global level function of non coding DNA.

Information Content

The 2.9 billion base pairs of the haploid human genome correspond to about 691.4 megabytes of data, since every base pair can be coded by 2 bits.

The entropy rate of the genome differs significantly between coding and non-coding sequences. It is close to the maximum of 2 bits per base pair for the coding sequences (about 45 million base pairs), but less for the non-coding parts. It ranges between 1.5 and 1.9 bits per base pair for the individual chromosome, except for the Y chromosome, which has an entropy rate below 0.9 bits per base pair.

Sequencing

DNA sequencing determines the order of the nucleotide bases in a genome.

Composite

The Human Genome Project and a parallel project by Celera Genomics each produced and published a haploid human genome sequence, both of which were a composite of the DNA sequence of several individuals.

Personal

A personal genome sequence is a complete sequencing of the chemical base pairs that make up the DNA of a single person. Because medical treatments have different effects on different people because of genetic variations such as single-nucleotide polymorphisms (SNPs), the analysis of personal genomes may lead to personalized medical treatment based on individual genotypes.

The completion of the fifth such map was announced in December 2008. The genome mapped was that of a Korean researcher Seong-Jin Kim. Genome maps had previously been completed for Craig Venter of the U.S. in 2007, James Watson of the U.S. in April 2008, and Yang Huanming of China in November 2008 and Dan Stoicescu in January 2008.

Personal genomes had not been sequenced in the Human Genome Project to protect the identity of volunteers who provided DNA samples.

That sequence was derived from the DNA of several volunteers from a diverse population. Another distinction is that the HGP sequence is haploid, however, the sequence maps for Venter and Watson for example are diploid, representing both sets of chromosomes.

Kim's genome had 1.58 million SNPs that had never been reported before and indicates that six out of 10,000 DNA bases are unique to Koreans. Kim's sequence map can be used to assist in building a standard Korean genome, which can then be used to compare the genomes of other Korean individuals for personalized medical treatments.

Mapping

Whereas a genome sequence lists the order of every DNA base in a genome, a genome map identifies the landmarks. A genome map is less detailed than a genome sequence and aids in navigating around the genome.

Variation

An example of a variation map is the HapMap being developed by the International HapMap Project. The HapMap is a haplotype map of the human genome, "which will describe the common patterns of human DNA sequence variation." It catalogs the patterns of small-scale variations in the genome that involve single DNA letters, or bases.

Researchers published the first sequence-based map of large-scale structural variation across the human genome in the journal *Nature* in May 2008. Large-scale structural variations are differences in the genome among people that range from a few thousand to a few million DNA bases; some are gains or losses of stretches of genome sequence and others appear as re-arrangements of stretches of sequence. These variations include differences in the number of copies individuals have of a particular gene, deletions, translocations and inversions.

Variation

Most studies of human genetic variation have focused on single-nucleotide polymorphisms (SNPs), which are substitutions in individual bases along a chromosome. Most analyses estimate that SNPs occur on average somewhere between every 1 in 100 and 1 in 300 base pairs in the euchromatic human genome, although they do not occur at a uniform density. Thus follows the popular statement that "we are all, regardless of race, genetically 99.9% the same", although this would be somewhat qualified by most geneticists. For example, a much larger fraction of the genome is now thought to be involved in copy number variation. A large-scale collaborative effort to catalogue SNP variations in the human genome is being undertaken by the International HapMap Project.

The genomic loci and length of certain types of small repetitive sequences are highly variable from person to person, which is the basis of DNA fingerprinting and DNA paternity testing technologies. The heterochromatic portions of the human genome, which total several hundred million base pairs, are also thought to be quite variable within the human population (they are so repetitive and so long that they cannot be accurately sequenced with current technology). These regions contain few genes, and it is unclear whether any significant phenotypic effect results from typical variation in repeats or heterochromatin.

Most gross genomic mutations in gamete germ cells probably result in inviable embryos; however, a number of human diseases are related to large-scale genomic abnormalities. Down syndrome, Turner Syndrome, and a number of other diseases result from nondisjunction of entire chromosomes. Cancer cells frequently have aneuploidy of chromosomes and chromosome arms, although a cause and effect relationship between aneuploidy and cancer has not been established.

Genetic Disorders

Most aspects of human biology involve both genetic (inherited) and non-genetic (environmental) factors. Some inherited variation influences aspects of our biology that are not medical in nature (height, eye colour, ability to taste or smell certain compounds, etc). Moreover, some genetic disorders only cause disease in combination with the appropriate environmental factors (such as diet). With these caveats, genetic disorders may be described as clinically defined diseases caused by genomic DNA sequence variation.

In the most straightforward cases, the disorder can be associated with variation in a single gene. For example, cystic fibrosis is caused by mutations in the CFTR gene, and is the most common recessive disorder in caucasian populations with over 1,300 different mutations known. Disease-causing mutations in specific genes are usually severe in terms of gene function, and are fortunately rare, thus genetic disorders are similarly individually rare. However, since there are many genes that can vary to cause genetic disorders, in aggregate they comprise a significant component of known medical conditions, especially in pediatric medicine. Molecularly characterized genetic disorders are those for which the underlying causal gene has been identified, currently there are approximately 2,200 such disorders annotated in the OMIM database.

Studies of genetic disorders are often performed by means of family-based studies. In some instances population based approaches are employed, particularly in the case of so-called founder populations such as those in Finland, French-Canada, Utah, Sardinia, etc. Diagnosis and treatment of genetic disorders are usually performed by a geneticist-physician trained in clinical/medical genetics. The results of the Human Genome Project are likely to provide increased availability of genetic testing for gene-related disorders, and eventually improved treatment. Parents can be screened for hereditary conditions and counselled on the consequences, the probability it will be inherited, and how to avoid or ameliorate it in their offspring. As noted above, there are many different kinds of DNA sequence variation, ranging from complete extra or missing chromosomes down to single nucleotide changes.

It is generally presumed that much naturally occurring genetic variation in human populations is phenotypically neutral, i.e. has little or no detectable effect on the physiology of the individual (although there may be fractional differences in fitness defined over evolutionary time frames). Genetic disorders can be caused by any or all known types of sequence variation. To molecularly characterize a new genetic disorder, it is necessary to establish a causal link between a particular genomic sequence variant and the clinical disease under investigation. Such studies constitute the realm of human molecular genetics.

With the advent of the Human Genome and International HapMap Project, it has become feasible to explore subtle genetic influences on many common disease conditions such as diabetes, asthma, migraine, schizophrenia, etc. Although some causal links have been made between genomic sequence variants in particular genes and some of these diseases, often with much publicity in the general media, these are usually not considered to be genetic disorders *per se* as their causes are complex, involving many different genetic and environmental factors. Thus there may be disagreement in particular cases whether a specific medical condition should be termed a genetic disorder.

Evolution

Comparative genomics studies of mammalian genomes suggest that approximately 5% of the human genome has been conserved by evolution since the divergence of extant lineages approximately 200 million years ago, containing the vast majority of genes.

Intriguingly, since genes and known regulatory sequences probably comprise less than 2% of the genome, this suggests that there may be more unknown functional sequence than known functional sequence. A smaller, yet substantial, fraction of human genes seem to be shared among most known vertebrates. The published chimpanzee genome differs from that of the human genome by 1.23% in direct sequence comparisons.

Around 20% of this figure is accounted for by variation within each species, leaving only ~1.06% consistent sequence divergence between humans and chimps at shared genes. This nucleotide by nucleotide difference is dwarfed, however, by the portion of each genome that is not shared, including around 6% of functional genes that are unique to either humans or chimps.

In other words, the considerable observable differences between humans and chimps may be due as much or more to genome level variation in the number, function and expression of genes rather than DNA sequence changes in shared genes. On average, a typical human protein-coding gene differs from its chimpanzee ortholog by only two amino acid substitutions; nearly one third of human genes have exactly the same protein translation as their chimpanzee orthologs. A major difference between the two genomes is human chromosome 2, which is equivalent to a fusion product of chimpanzee chromosomes 12 and 13 (later renamed to chromosomes 2A and 2B, respectively).

Humans have undergone an extraordinary loss of olfactory receptor genes during our recent evolution, which explains our relatively crude sense of smell compared to most other mammals. Evolutionary evidence suggests that the emergence of colour vision in humans and several other primate species has diminished the need for the sense of smell.

Chimpanzee Genome Project

The Chimpanzee Genome Project is an effort to determine the DNA sequence of the Chimpanzee genome. It is expected that by comparing the genomes of humans and other apes, it will be possible to better understand what makes humans distinct from other species.

Chimp-human chromosome differences. The major structural difference is that human chromosome 2 (green colour code) was derived from two smaller chromosomes that are found in other great apes. Parts of human chromosome 2 are scattered among parts of several cat and rat chromosomes in these species that are more distantly related to humans (more ancient common ancestors; about 85 million years since the human/rodent common ancestor: Entrez Pubmed 12552136)

Identification of Human Chromsome

The recognition of chromosome bonds has provided new morphologic features for use in the identification of human chromosomes and chromosomal parts. In addition to the telomere, centromere, and arms, special landmarks (*i.e.*, well-defined bands) were selected to subdivides the arms into regions. The regions are designaled 1,2,3, and 4, moving from the centromere towards the telomere. Using the nomenclater established at the Paris conference is 1971, any particular band or segment of a chromosome can be identified according to the following parameters:

- Chromosome number,
- An arm symbol (p=short arm, q=long),
- The region and band numbers.

For example, 6p23 indicates band number 3 in region 2 of the short arm of chromosome 6. With the use of the banding techniques, particularly the G and Q banding some 320 bands per haploid set can be identified at metaphase. However, if mitosis of followed through late prophase and prometaphase, up to 1256 bands may be recognized.

Determination of Sex

The well-known fact that male and female individuals are statistically found in about equal members suggests that sex is determined by a hereditary mechanism There is physiology and cytologic proof that sex is determined as soon as the egg is fertilized and that it depends on the gametes. Among the physiology evidence is the finding that identical twins—which originate from a single zygote—are always of the same sex. Cytologic evidence was first obtained by McClug, who demonstrated that the karyorpe of a cell is composed not only of common chromosomes (*autosomes*) but also of one or more special chromosomes that are distinguished from the autosomes by morphologic characteristics and behaviour: These were called *accessory chromosomes, allosomes, heterochromsomes, of sex chromosomes.*

The majority of organisms have a pair of sex chromsome, which in the course of evolution, have been specialized for sex determination. One of the sexes has a pair of identical sex chromosomes (XX); the other may have a single sex chromosome, which may be unpaired (XO) or paired with a Y chromosome (XY) The XY pair is also called *hetermorphic* because of the different morphology of the chromosomes.

In the human the garments are not identical with respect to the sex chromosomes. The male is heterozygous (XY) and produces two types of spermatozoa in similar proportions, *i.e.,* one carries the X chromosome, and the other the Y. the female, being homozygous (XX), produces only one kind of gamete (the ovum). Therefore only two combinations of gametes are possible at fertilization and the result is 50 per cent males and 50 per cent females. This type of sex determination is found in all mammals and in certain insects, such as *Drosophila.* In other vertebrates and certain invertebrates, the female is heterogametic, and the male, homogametic. In some animals the sex chromosomes cannot be distinguished from the other. In such cases the sexdetermining genes are confined to a region in a pair of chromosomes.

In the human the Y chromosome contains an essential testis-determining factor and determines the male sex. The genes involved are situated in a region near the centromere. An individual with XO (lacking the Y chromosome) will resemble a female but will have atrophied ovaries (Turner's syndrome).

We have seen earlier that the X and Y chromosomes differ in size and morphology. In the XY pair there is a *homologous region* in which recombination may take place during meiosis and a *differential region* that is unpaired.

Interphase Nuclei

The X chromatin can be bound as a small body in different positions within the nucleus. For example, in nerve cells it may be near the nucleolus in the nucleoplasm, or near the nuclear envelope.

In cells of the oral mucosa it is generally attached to the envelope, and in neutrophil leukocytes it may appear as a small rod called the *drumstick.*

The study of sex chromatin has a wide field of medical applications and offers the possibility of relating the origin of certain congenital diseases to chromosome anomalies. Among these application is the diagnosis of sex in intersexual states in postnatal and even in fetal life. The frequency with which sex chromation can be detected in the female varies from tissue to tissue. In nervous tissue the frequency may be 85 per cent, whereas in whole mounts of amniotic or chorionic epithelium it may be as high as 96 per cent. In oral smears the frequency may vary between 20 and 50 per cent in normal females.

The differential behaviour of the two X chromosome in the female led Lyon to the so-called *inactive* X *hypothesis* is genetically active; the X undergoing heteropyknosis may be either of maternal or paternal origin, and the decision by which X becomes inactive is taken at random; the inactivation occures early in embryonic life and remains fixed. It is now admitted that only a part of the X chromosome condenses into a Barr corpuscle; This condensed chromosome is said to contain *facultative heterochromatin,* as opposed to the *constitutive heterochromatin* found in other chromosome takes place even in 3X and 4X individuals, in which only one X remains uncondensed.

The inactivation starts in the human in the late blastocyst stage on about the sixteenth day of embryonic life; the inactivated X chromosome then remains heterochromatic in the somatic cells.

The fact that X inactivation occurs at random has been demonstrated in human diseases linked to the X chromosome. The *Lesch-Nyhansyndrome,* in which a deficiency of one enzyme of the purine metabolism (*i.e.,* hypoxanthine-guanine phosphoribosyl transferase) produces mental retardation and increase uric acid levels, results from a recessive mutation in the X chromsome. When fibroblasts of heterozygous women are cultured in vitro, two types of cell clones are obtained. Half the clones contain the enzyme, whereas the other half lack the enzyme.

During the cell cycle the heterochromatic X chromosome is characterized by its late replication. This can be clearly observed by the use of 5-bromodeoxyuridine, followed by the fluorescent dye. Hoechst 33258 or the Giemsa stain.

The above-mentioned fluorescence method for the study of Q banding led to the demonstration of that a large portion of the Y chromosome is heterochromatic and appears, at interphase, as a strongly fluorescent body, the so- called Y *chromatin*. While the X chromatin is 1.0 to 1.2 μm in diameter, the Y chromatin is only about 0.7-μm in diameter and generally is not attached to the nuclear envelope.

The number of Y chromation bodies is identical to the number of Y chromosome. For example, individuals with XYY have two Y chromatin bodies. The human Y chromosome consists of two segments, one that does not fluoresce and is genetically active. and a second that fluoresces and is genetically inactive. It is this latter segment that may be polymorphic, showing wide variations in size between individuals. Among mammal, only man and the gorilla share this fluorescent region of the Y chromosome, suggesting that it is of recent evolutionalry origin.

This region corresponds to a highly repetitive (satellite) DNA, which is specific fore the Y chromosome and probably has no genetic function.

Although the primary determination of sex is made at fertilization the embryo acquires its definite sex characteristics by a more complex mechanism. An epigenetic factor (*i.e.*, hormonal) may assume control of the genetic determination during development, thereby changing the phenotypic direction of sex. Among vertebrates a condition of bisexuality may exist (*e.g.*, the coexistence of structures of the functional sex, together with primordia of the heterologous sex). For example, male amphibians have a redimentary ovary (Bidder's organ) and vestigial oviducts.

In the human embryo until the sixth week the gonads and the primordia of the urogenital tract are identical in males and females. At this time the gonad has already has already been invaded by the primary XX or XY germ cells. At this point, a gene (or set of genes) present in the y chromosome causes the undifferentiated gonad to differentiate into a testis, and the absence of this gene allows the gonad to become an ovary. The development into a testis, and the absence of this gene allows the gonad to become an ovary.

The development into a testis starts as soon as the *gonocytes* (*i.e.*, primordial germ cells) from the yolk sac have finished their migration into the *gonadal ridge*. Gonocytes of the male (XY) migrate deeper into the gonadal blastema, and female gonocytes (XX) remain at the periphery, forming a thick cortical layer.

H-Y Antigen

It is known that the Y chromosome directs the organogenesis of the testis by inducing the production of a protein (or membrane and determines, by cell recognition, the formation of the seminiferous tubule. It has been proposed that a Y-linked determining gene of mammals produces that a Y-linked determining gene of mammals produces this *H-T antigen,* which is found in various cell types in males but is absent in females.

This antigen is also a histocompatibility factor (H) that is found, for example, in the skin of male mice and that determines the rejection of female skin transplants.

Action of Testosterone

The gonad differentiates into a definite testicle at the seventh week, whereas the female gonad differentiates between the eighth and ninth weeks of development, At the time of differentiation an important epigenetic factor is the production of androgens by somatic cells in the embryonic male gonad.

In mammals administration of *testosterone* (the male hormone) to the mother produces in the fetus a shift in the differentiation of XX genitalia to a male type, producting what is called *feminine masculine pseudohermaphroditism*. This hormone acting locally accelerates the development of the testis, whereas in the female the absence of the hormone permits the slower development characteristic of the ovary.

Chromosomal Abnormalities

The study of chromosome abnormalities in man, like that of normal cytogenetics, can be divided into periods before and after the development of the banding techniques. In the earlier period it was found that 0.5 per cent of all newborns have gross chromosomal abnormalities, about half of which are in the sex chromosomes and the rest of which are in the autosomes. These abnormalities generally consist of aneuploidy, such as monosomy or trisomy, Structural aberrations, such as translocation, deficiency, duplication, and other more complex alterations, have also been observed;

Diagnosis of chromosomal aberrations can be made even before a child is born. This is done by removing amitotic fluid by puncturing the mother's abdomen, a procedure called *amniocentesis. which* does not entail risks to the fetus. The amniotic fluid contains cells shed from the fetus and which can be cultured.

This technique is useful for karyotyping the babies off mothers with a history of chromosomal abnormality, or children of those who are carriers of a balanced translocation, in whom that risk of conceiving an affected child is high. In addition, this technique permits the *antenatal* determination of the fetal sex, which may be of importance in certain sex-linked diseases.

The improved resolution provided by the banding techniques has not only confirmed the previously observed abnormalities but has also led to the discovery of over 30 new chromosomal syndromes and several malignancies defects.

In aneuploidy the genetic message contained in each chromosome is maintained intact. The alteration is quantitative; it resides in a disequilibrium established by the excess (trisomy) or deficit (monosomy) in the amount of genetic material, Such a dosage effect may be dangerous to the organism and may produce severe anatomical and functional anomalies (*i.e.*, malformations). It will be shown later that trisomy produces changes that are characteristic for each chromosome present in excess; however, in all instances of trisomy the tendency is towards involution of the nervous system, resulting in a more or less severe mental defect.

Another important consequence of aneuploidy is spontaneous abortion. A large proportion of aborted fetuses show trisomy in one of the larger chromosomes in the karyotype. Aneuploidy of one the larger chromosomes is generally lethal, being more severe than an equivalent alteration in a smaller chromosome. Malformation mental retardation, sterility, and spontaneously abortion operate as strong selective mechanisms tending to eliminate from the general population those individuals carrying deleterious genetic imbalances.

Aneuploidy originates by the mechanism called *Non-disjunction.* The immediate cause of non-disjuction is the lagging, during anaphase, of one sister chromatid which during telophase remains in one of the cells together with the other sister chromatid. This change gives rise to a cell line that lacks one chromosome or has one chromosome in excess for that pair (monosomy and trisomy).

Non-disjunction may occur during *meiosis, giving* rise to an aneuploid *ovum. This* when fertilized by a normal spermatozoon, results in a zygote and later an organism in which all cells are aneuploid. In some cases the alteration may be in the male gamete or in both, thus producing more complex types of abnormalities. If non-disjunction occurs in a *mitotic division,* which precedes the formation of germ cells, the effects are similar to those of *meiotic non-disjunction.* If mitotic non-disjunction occurs during embryonic development, a *mosaic* of different cell lines is produced.

We mentioned earlier the various structural aberrations that are found in human chromosomes (*i.e.,* translocation, deficiency, and duplication). The most common of these is the so-called *reciprocal translocation,* in which chromosome segments are exchanged between non-homologous chromosomes. Some of these translocations may result in a chromosome having a length and configuration that may be easily identified. However, in other cases the apparent morphology changes very little. Banding techniques are of fundamental importance in detecting such cases. The most important aberrations or as follows.

Klinefelter's Syndrome

Most affected individuals are practically normal except for minor phenotypic anomalies. They have small testes, frequent gynecomastia (enlarged breasts), tendency to tallness, obesity and underdevelopment of secondary sex characteristics. Spermatogenesis does not occur, thereby resulting in complete infertility. These individuals have a positive sex chromatin and 47 chromosomes (44 autosomes + XXY). Males with 48 chromosome (44 autosome+XXXY) and two Barr corpuscles have also been described. These individuals have features of klinefelter's syndrome and are mentally retarded. Persons with 49 chromosomes (44 autosomes+XXXXY) have also been reported. They display extensive skeletal anomalies, extreme hypogenitalism, and severe mental deficiency. These persons have three X chromation bodies.

XYY Syndrome

Males having two Y chromosomes have been identified in the past in maximum security institutions. It was proposed that such individuals had a strong tendency to ward anti-social behaviour and aggression. More recently, XYY individuals have been found in the normal population in a proportion of 1 in `650 male infants, suggesting that the correlation with violence may not be a strong as was previously thought.

Gonadal Dysgenesis

Patients with Turner's syndrome usually have a female appearance with short stature, webbed neck (folds of skin extended from the mastoid to the shoulders) and generally infantile internal sexual organs. The ovary does not develop and shows complete absence of germ cells. As result of this ovarian dysgenesis, menstruation does not occur, and secondary sexual characteristics do not develop.

The karyotype shows 45 chromosomes (44 autosomes +X), and there is no sexchromation. In this syndrome there is little difference in the gonads up to the third moth of gestation; the ovaries up to the third month of gestation; the ovaries contain approximately the normal number of germ cells (about 2 or 3×10^6 cells) later on there is a rapid atresia of the germ cells, leading to their virtually disappearance after puberty. It is probable that the lack of one X chromosomes determines the progressive ovarian atresia by failure of primordial follicles.

Females with X Polysomy

Triplo-X constitution (47 chromosome; 44 autosomes + XXX) was detected in phenotypically near-normal females. A number of these females are mentally subnormal or psychotic and some of them menstruate. The sex chromatin bodies are found in cells from these women. A few severely retarded patients with three corpuscles of sex chromatin and 48 chromosomes (44 autosomes + XXXX) have been found. These persons are also called metafermales Mixed Chromosomal Aberrations. Kinefelter's syndrome may be found combined with mongolism. Such a person has 48 chromosomes: 45 autosomes (including a trisomic pair 21) +XXY.

Mosaics

Sometimes chromsomal aberrations are produced during development of the embryo. One interesing example is induced by the loss of one Y chromosomes in the first division of the zygote. This may result in twins, of which one has normal male characters and the other has Tuner's syndrome. Sometimes chromosomal aberrations due to non-disjunction are produced during development of the embryo. These individuals possess different chromosomal complements from cell to cell within the same tissue or between tissues, depending on the embryonic stage at which non-disjunction occurred.

Hermaphroditism

A true hermaphrodite is an individual who has both ovarian and testicular tissue. The two types of gonadal tissue may be separated or in close proximity (ovotestis). Frequently, true hermaphrodites haves a 46, XX chromosome complement and are chromation-positive. Other may have a 46, XY mosaicism has also been detected in this condition.

Mongolism

Before the development of the banding techniques about 12 classic syndromes had been described, the majority of which were caused by an extra chromosome or loss of a chromsome segment. Except for the X monosomy (Turner's syndrome), any other monosomy is believed to be inviable (*i.e.*, leads to death of the embryo). This also holds true for all trisomies other than those of chromosomes 13, 18, or 21.

21-Monosomy

Complete deletion of one of the chromosomes in pair 21 is apparently lethal, but there is a syndrome in which a large part of cone is lacking. Children with this condition have a morphologic aspect which is, to some extent, the opposite of mongolism. The nose is prominent, the distance between eyes shorter than normal, and the ears are large and the muscles contracted, It seems that in trisomy and monosomy of the 21st, the phenotype shifts to one or the other side of normal.

18-Trisomy

In this case the child is small and weak, the head is laterally flattened, and the helix of the ear scarcely developed. The hands are short and the digital imprints are rather simple. These children are very retarded mentally and usually die before one year of age.

18-Monosomy

This is the opposite syndrome is which a partial deletion of one chromosome of the pair occures. The ears are voluminous, the fingers long, and the digital imprints are complex and convoluted.

21-Trisomy Mongolism

Among the most important autosomal aberrations is *mongolism*, which is characterized by multiple malformations, mental retardation, and markedly defective development of the central nervous system. It was discovered that the mongoloid has an extra chromosome. Pair 21 is trisomic instead of normal. This aberration probably originates from non-disjunction of pair 21 during meiosis.

The extra chromosome of pair 21 in some cases may become attached to another autosome (translocation), usually to pair 22. The phenotype of a mongoloid is recognizable at birth in most cases. The face of such a patient has a special moon-like aspect, with oblique palpebral fissures, increased separation between the eyes, and a skin fold (epicanthus) at the inner part of the eyes. The nose is flattened the ears and the tongue protrudes.

Mongolism is the most common congenital disease and is present in more than 0.1 per cent of births. Its frequency increases as the mother's age sporadic and in general there is no recurrence in the family. However, in the rarer cases of mongolism by translocation, the disease may affect siblings and may appear in successive generation. Fortunately this "translocation trisomy" represents only 3 to 4 per cent of all call cases of mongolism. In this type there is no change in frequency with the age of the mother, and when the aberration is properly determined by karyotype analysis, the parents should be warned of a repetition of this defect.

13-Trisomy

Multiple and severe body malformations, as well as profound mental deficiency, are characteristic features. The head is small and the eyes are often small, or absent. are-lip, cleft palate, and malformations of the brain are frequent. The internal organs are also severely malformed and in most cases death occurs soon after birth.

One of the most remarkable phenotypes associated with a chromosome structural change is the condition known as *cri du chat* syndrome. The affected baby has a strange mewing cry, multiple malfomations and mental retardation associated with partial deletion of the short arm of chromosome 5. Another type of patient showing facial alteration and skeletal and ophthalmologic abnormalities along with profound mental retadation, is the carrier of a deletion of the long arm of chromosome 18.

The use of the banding techniques has permitted the detection of more than 30 new chromosomal syndromes which result from a partial trisomy or deletion from each of almost all the chromosome.

Such alterations have been bound in children with mental retardation or minor congenital defects and also in some with normal intelligence and minor anomalies which were earlier considered as deviations of normality. The technical advances have permitted the identification of chromosome defects even when there are few clinical symptoms furthermore, these methods have allowed the study of cases of balanced chromosomal translocations, which, as carriers of this type of syndrome, are important to detect. In such cases transmission can be prevented by proper counselling and prenatal diagnosis.

Chromosomal Aberrations

The development of the banding techniques has also resulted in the demonstration of specific chromosomal defects in certain types of tymors. Here only a few examples will be given. The most characteristic of these is the association of *chronic myelogenous leukemia* with the so-called *Philadelphia chromosome* (Ph 1). This involves a balanced translocation between chromosome 9 and 22. The Ph 1 chromosome is acquired with the disease and is not found in cultured fifbroblasts or in the idential twins of affected patients. In a *retinoblastoma* (*i.e.*, a cancer of the retina) a deletion in the long arm of chromosomes 13 has been identified. Other abnormalities have been observed in lymphomas, meingiomas, and many other tumors. Cancer cells are usually associated with severe chromosomal abnormalities such as polyploidy and aneuploidy.

Starting the Chimpanzee Genome Project

Human and chimpanzee chromosomes are very similar. The primary difference is that humans have one fewer pair of chromosomes than do other great apes. Humans have 23 pairs of chromosomes and other great apes have 24 pairs of chromosomes. In the human evolutionary lineage, two ancestral ape chromosomes fused at their telomeres producing human chromosome 2. There are nine other major chromosomal differences between chimpanzees and humans: chromosome segment inversions on human chromosomes 1, 4, 5, 9, 12, 15, 16, 17, and 18.

After the completion of the Human genome project, a Common Chimpanzee genome project was initiated. In December 2003, a preliminary analysis of 7600 genes shared between the two genomes confirmed that certain genes such as the forkhead-box P2 transcription factor, which is involved in speech development, are different in the human lineage. Several genes involved in hearing were also found to have changed during human evolution, suggesting selection involving human language-related Behaviour. Differences between individual humans and Common Chimpanzees are estimated to be about 10 times the typical difference between pairs of humans.

Draft Genome Sequence of the Common Chimpanzee

Analysis of the genome was published in *Nature* on September 1, 2005, in an article produced by the Chimpanzee Sequencing and Analysis Consortium, a group of scientists which is supported in part by the National Human Genome Research Institute, one of the National Institutes of Health.

The article marked the completion of the draft genome sequence. A database now exists containing the genetic differences between human and chimpanzee genes, with about thirty-five million single-nucleotide changes, five million insertion/deletion events, and various chromosomal rearrangements. Gene duplications account for most of the sequence differences between humans and chimps. Single-base-pair substitutions account for about half as much genetic change as does gene duplication.

Typical human and chimp homologs of proteins differ in only an average of two amino acids. About 30 percent of all human proteins are identical in sequence to the corresponding chimp protein. As mentioned above, gene duplications are a major source of differences between human and chimp genetic material, with about 2.7 percent of the genome now representing differences having been produced by gene duplications or deletions during approximately 6 million years since humans and chimps diverged from their common evolutionary ancestor. The comparable variation within human populations is 0.5 percent.

About 600 genes have been identified that may have been undergoing strong positive selection in the human and chimp lineages; many of these genes are involved in immune system defence against microbial disease or are targeted receptors of pathogenic microorganisms (example: Glycophorin C and *Plasmodium falciparum*). By comparing human and chimp genes to the genes of other mammals, it has been found that genes coding for transcription factors, such as forkhead-box P2 (FOXP2), have often evolved faster in the human relative to chimp; relatively small changes in these genes may account for the morphological differences between humans and chimps. A set of 348 transcription factor genes code for proteins with an average of about 50 percent more amino acid changes in the human lineage than in the chimp lineage.

Six human chromosomal regions were found that may have been under particularly strong and coordinated selection during the past 250,000 years. These regions contain at least one marker allele that seems unique to the human lineage while the entire chromosomal region shows lower than normal genetic variation. This pattern suggests that one or a few strongly selected genes in the chromosome region may have been preventing the random accumulation of neutral changes in other nearby genes.

One such region on chromosome 7 contains the FOXP2 gene (mentioned above) and this region also includes the Cystic fibrosis transmembrane conductance regulator (CFTR) gene, which is important for ion transport in tissues such as the salt-secreting epithelium of sweat glands. Human mutations in the CFTR gene might be selected for as a way to survive cholera.

Another such region on chromosome 4 may contain elements regulating the expression of a nearby protocadherin gene that may be important for brain development and function. Although changes in expression of genes that are expressed in the brain tend to be less than for other organs (such as liver) on average, gene expression changes in the brain have been more dramatic in the human lineage than in the chimp lineage. This is consistent with the dramatic divergence of the unique pattern of human brain development seen in the human lineage compared to the ancestral great ape pattern. The protocadherin-beta gene cluster on chromosome 5 also shows evidence of possible positive selection.

Results from the human and chimp genome analyses should help in understanding some human diseases. Humans appear to have lost a functional caspase-12 gene, which in other primates codes for an enzyme that may protect against Alzheimer's disease. Figures published in *Nature* on September 1, 2005, in an article produced by the Chimpanzee Sequencing and Analysis Consortium, show that 24% of the chimpanzee genome does not align with the human genome. There are 3% further alignment gaps, 1.23% SNP differences, and 2.7% copy number variations totaling at least 30% differences between chimpanzee and *Homo sapiens* genomes.

Genes of the Chromosome 2 Fusion Site

The results of the chimpanzee genome project suggest that when ancestral chromosomes 2A and 2B fused to produce human chromosome 2, no genes were lost from the fused ends of 2A and 2B. At the site of fusion, there are approximately 150,000 base pairs of sequence not found in chimpanzee chromosomes 2A and 2B. Additional linked copies of the PGML/FOXD/CBWD genes exist elsewhere in the human genome, particularly near the p end of chromosome 9.

This suggests that a copy of these genes may have been added to the end of the ancestral 2A or 2B prior to the fusion event. It remains to be determined if these inserted genes confer a selective advantage.

- PGML. The phosphoglucomutase-like gene of human chromosome 2. This gene is incomplete and may not produce a functional transcript.

- FOXD. The forkhead box D4-like gene is an example of an intronless gene. The function of this gene is not known, but it may code for a transcription control protein.

- CBWD. Cobalamin synthetase is a bacterial enzyme that makes vitamin B_{12}. In the distant past, a common ancestor to mice and apes incorporated a copy of a cobalamin synthetase gene. Humans are unusual in that they have several copies of cobalamin synthetase-like genes, including the one on chromosome 2. It remains to be determined what the function of these human cobalamin synthetase-like genes is. If these genes are involved in vitamin B_{12} metabolism, this could be relevant to human evolution. A major change in human development is greater post-natal brain growth than is observed in other apes. Vitamin B_{12} is important for brain development, and vitamin B_{12} deficiency during brain development results in severe neurological defects in human children.

- CXYorf1-like protein. Several transcripts of unknown function corresponding to this region have been isolated. This region is also present in the closely related chromosome 9p terminal region that contains copies of the PGML/FOXD/CBWD genes.

- Many ribosomal protein L23a pseudogenes are scattered through the human genome.

Mitochondrial Genome

The human mitochondrial genome, while usually not included when referring to the "human genome", is of tremendous interest to geneticists, since it undoubtedly plays a role in mitochondrial disease. It also sheds light on human evolution; for example, analysis of variation in the human mitochondrial genome has led to the postulation of a recent common ancestor for all humans on the maternal line of descent.

Due to the lack of a system for checking for copying errors, Mitochondrial DNA (mtDNA) has a more rapid rate of variation than nuclear DNA. This 20-fold increase in the mutation rate allows mtDNA to be used for more accurate tracing of maternal ancestry. Studies of mtDNA in populations have allowed ancient migration paths to be traced, such as the migration of Native Americans from Siberia or Polynesians from southeastern Asia. It has also been used to show that there is no trace of Neanderthal DNA in the European gene mixture inherited through purely maternal lineage.

Epigenome

Epigenetics are a variety of features of the human genome that transcend its primary DNA sequence, such as chromatin packaging, histone modifications and DNA methylation, and which are important in regulating gene expression, genome replication and other cellular processes. Epigenetic markers strengthen and weaken transcription of certain genes but do not affect the actual sequence of DNA nucleotides.

Craig Venter # Individual Human Genome Sequenced

John Craig Venter (born October 14, 1946) is an American biologist and entrepreneur, most famous for his role in being one of the first to sequence the human genome and for his role in creating the first cell with a synthetic genome in 2010. Venter founded Celera Genomics, The Institute for Genomic Research and the J. Craig Venter Institute, now working at the latter to create synthetic biological organisms and to document genetic diversity in the world's oceans. He was listed on *Time* magazine's 2007 and 2008 Time 100 list of the most influential people in the world. In 2010, The British Magazine New Statesman listed Craig Venter at 14th in the list of "The World's 50 Most Influential Figures 2010".

Early Life

Venter was born in Salt Lake City, Utah. In his youth, Venter did not take his education seriously, preferring to spend his time on the water in boats or surfing. According to his biography, *A Life Decoded*, he was said to never be a terribly engaged student, having Cs and Ds on his eighth-grade report cards. According to *Time Magazine*, it was not always evident that Venter would become a transformative figure, particularly when he was a boy.

Although he was against the Vietnam War, Venter was drafted and enlisted in the United States Navy where he worked in the intensive-care ward of a field hospital. Being confronted with wounded, maimed, and dying soldiers on a daily basis instilled in him a desire to study medicine — although he later switched to scientific medical research.

Education

Venter graduated from Mills High School and began his college career at a community college, College of San Mateo in California. He received his B.S. degree in biochemistry in 1972, and his Ph.D. degree in physiology and pharmacology in 1975, both from the University of California, San Diego. At UCSD, he studied under biochemist Nathan O. Kaplan, and married former Ph.D. candidate Barbara Rae.

After working as an associate professor, and later as full professor, at the State University of New York at Buffalo, he joined the National Institutes of Health in 1984. In Buffalo, he divorced Dr. Rae-Venter and married his student, Claire M. Fraser, remaining married to her until 2005.

Discovery

While at the NIH, Venter learned of a technique for rapidly identifying all of the mRNAs present in a cell and began to use it to identify human brain genes. The short cDNA sequence fragments discovered by this method are called expressed sequence tags (ESTs) a name coined by Anthony Kerlavage at The Institute for Genomic Research. The NIH initially led an effort to patent these gene fragments, in which Venter coincidentally and controversially became involved. The NIH later withdrew the patent applications, following public outcry. Subsequent court cases declared that ESTs were not directly patentable.

Human Genome Project

Venter was passionate about the power of genomics to radically transform healthcare. Venter believed that shotgun sequencing was the fastest and most effective way to get useful human genome data. The method was controversial, however, since some geneticists felt it would not be accurate enough for a genome as complicated as that of humans. Frustrated with what Venter viewed as the slow pace of progress in the Human Genome project, and unable to get funds for his ideas, he sought funding from the private sector to fund Celera Genomics.

The goal of the company was to sequence the entire human genome and release it into the public domain for non-commercial use in much less time and for much less cost than the public human genome project. The company planned to monetize their work by creating a value-added database of genomic data to which users could subscribe for a fee.

The goal consequently put pressure on the public genome program and spurred several groups to redouble their efforts to produce the full sequence. DNA from five demographically different individuals was used by Celera to generate the sequence of the human genome; one of the individuals was Venter himself. In 2000, Venter and Francis Collins of the National Institutes of Health and U.S. Public Genome Project jointly made the announcement of the mapping of the human genome in 2000, a full three years ahead of the expected end of the Public Genome Program.

The announcement was made along with US President Bill Clinton, and U.K. Prime Minister Tony Blair. Venter and Collins thus shared an award for "Biography of the Year" from A&E Network. Celera published the first Human Genome in the journal Science, and was soon followed by a Human Genome Project Publication in Nature. Despite some claims that shotgun sequencing was in some ways less accurate than the clone-by-clone method chosen by the Human Genome Project, the technique became widely accepted by the scientific community and is still the de facto standard used today.

Although Celera was originally set to sequence a composite of DNA samples, partway through the sequencing, Venter switched the samples for his own DNA. After contributing to the Human Genome, and its release it into the public domain, Venter was fired by Celera in early 2002. According to his biography, Venter was ready to leave Celera, and was fired due to conflict with the main investor, Tony White, that had existed since day one of the project. Venter writes that his main goal was always to accelerate science and thereby discovery, and he only sought help from the corporate world when he couldn't find funding in the public sector.

Ocean Sampling

The Global Ocean Sampling Expedition (GOS) is an ocean exploration genome project with the goal of assessing the genetic diversity in marine microbial communities and to understand their role in nature's fundamental processes. Begun as a Sargasso Sea pilot sampling project in August 2003, Craig Venter announced the full Expedition on 4 March 2004. The project, which used Craig Venter's personal yacht, *Sorcerer II*, started in Halifax, Canada, circumnavigated the globe and returned to the U.S. in January 2006.

Current Work

Venter is currently the president of the J. Craig Venter Institute, which conducts research in synthetic biology. In June 2005, he co-founded Synthetic Genomics, a firm dedicated to using modified microorganisms to produce clean fuels and biochemicals. In July 2009, ExxonMobil announced a $600 million collaboration with Synthetic Genomics to research and develop next-generation biofuels.

Venter is a member of the USA Science and Engineering Festival's Advisory Board.

Media Coverage

Venter has been the subject of articles in several magazines, including *Wired*, *The Economist*, Australian science magazine *Cosmos*, and *The Atlantic*. Additionally, he was featured on *The Colbert Report* on both February 27, 2007, and October 30, 2007.

Venter appeared in the "Evolution" episode of the documentary television series *Understanding*.

On May 16, 2004, Venter gave the commencement speech at Boston University.

In a 2007 interview with *New Scientist* when asked "Assuming you can make synthetic bacteria, what will you do with them?", Venter replied:

Over the next 20 years, synthetic genomics is going to become the standard for making anything. The chemical industry will depend on it. Hopefully, a large part of the energy industry will depend on it. We really need to find an alternative to taking carbon out of the ground, burning it, and putting it into the atmosphere. That is the single biggest contribution I could make.

Furthermore it suggests that one of the main purposes for creating synthetic bacteria would be to reduce the dependence on fossil fuels through bioremediation.

On May 10, 2007, Venter was awarded an honorary doctorate from Arizona State University., and on October 24 of the same year, he received an honorary doctorate from Imperial College London.

He was on the 2007 Time 100 most influential people in the world list made by Time magazine. In 2007 he also received the Golden Eurydice Award for contributions to Biophilosophy.

On September 4, 2007, a team led by Venter published the first complete (six-billion-letter) genome of an individual human — Venter's own DNA sequence. When on BBC News on October 22, 2007, when asked about his religious view he replied that he thought that a true scientist could not believe in supernatural explanations.

On December 4, 2007, Venter gave the Dimbleby lecture for the BBC in London. He outlined his current work and future developments in genetics.

In February 2008, he gave a speech about his current work at the TED conference.

Venter delivered the 2008 convocation speech for Faculty of Science honours and specialization students at the University of Alberta. A transcription of the speech is available here.

Dr. Venter was featured in Time Magazine's "The Top 10 Everything of 2008" article. Number three in 2008's Top 10 Scientific Discoveries was a piece outlining his work stitching together the 582,000 base pairs necessary to invent the genetic information for a whole new bacterium.

Dr. Venter took part in the inaugural San Diego Science Festival and spoke at its press conference on February 26, 2009.

On April 6, 2009, Venter gave a speech at Arizona State University as part of the Origins Symposium.

For an episode aired on July 27, 2009, Venter was interviewed on his boat by BBC One for the first episode of TV show Bang Goes the Theory.

On May 20, 2010, Venter announced the creation of first self-replicating synthetic bacterial cell.

On November 21, 2010 Steve Kroft profiled J. Craig Venter and his research on 60 minutes.

Individual Human Genome Sequenced

On September 4, 2007, a team led by Sam Levy published the first complete (six-billion-letter) genome of an individual human—Venter's own DNA sequence. Some of the sequences in Venter's genome are associated with wet earwax, increased risk of antisocial Behaviour, Alzheimer's and cardiovascular diseases. This publication was especially interesting since it contained a diploid instead of a haploid genome and shows promise for personalized medicine via genotyping. This genome, rather immodestly dubbed HuRef by Levy et al., was a landmark accomplishment and as of mid-2010 is probably the highest quality personal genome sequence yet completed.

The Human Reference Genome Browser is a web application for the navigation and analysis of Venter's recently published genome. The HuRef database consists of approximately 32 million DNA reads sequenced using microfluidic Sanger sequencing, assembled into 4,528 scaffolds and 4.1 million DNA variations identified by genome analysis. These variants include single-nucleotide polymorphisms (SNPs), block substitutions, short and large indels, and structural variations like insertions, deletions, inversions and copy number changes.

The browser enables scientists to navigate the HuRef genome assembly and sequence variations, and to compare it with the NCBI human build 36 assembly in the context of the NCBI and Ensembl annotations. The browser provides a comparative view between NCBI and HuRef consensus sequences, the sequence multi-alignment of the HuRef assembly, Ensembl and dbSNP annotations, HuRef variants, and the underlying variant evidence and functional analysis. The interface also represents the haplotype blocks from which diploid genome sequence can be inferred and the relation of variants to gene annotations. The display of variants and gene annotations are linked to external public resources including dbSNP, Ensembl, Online Mendelian Inheritance in Man (OMIM) and Gene Ontology (GO).

Users can search the HuRef genome using HUGO gene names, Ensembl and dbSNP identifiers, HuRef contig or scaffold locations, or NCBI chromosome locations. Users can then easily and quickly browse any genomic region via the simple and intuitive pan and zoom controls; furthermore, data relevant to specific loci can be exported for further analysis.

Mycoplasma Laboratorium

Venter is seeking to patent the first life form created by humanity, possibly to be named *Mycoplasma laboratorium*. There is speculation that this line of research could lead to producing bacteria that have been engineered to perform specific reactions, e.g. produce fuels, make medicines, combat global warming, etc.

In May 2010, a team of scientists led by Venter became the first to successfully create what was described as "synthetic life". This was done by synthesizing a very long DNA molecule containing an entire bacterium genome, and introducing this into another cell, analogous to the accomplishment of Eckard Wimmer's group, who synthesized and ligated an RNA virus genome and "booted" it in cell lysate. The single-celled organism contains four "watermarks" written into its DNA to identify it as synthetic and to help trace its descendants. The watermarks include

1. Code table for entire alphabet with punctuations
2. Names of 46 contributing scientists
3. Three quotations
4. The web address for the cell.

Genetic Distance

Genetic distance refers to the genetic divergence between species or between populations within a species. It considers a variety of parameters used to measure the genetic distance. Smaller genetic distances indicate a close genetic relationship whereas large genetic distances indicate a more distant genetic relationship. Genetic distance can be used to compare the genetic similarity between different species, such as humans and chimpanzees. Within a species genetic distance can be used to measure the divergence between different sub-species.

In its simplest form, the genetic distance between two populations is the difference in frequencies of a trait. For example the frequency of RH negative individuals is 50.4% among Basques, 41.2% in France and 41.1% in England. Thus the genetic difference between the Basques and French is 9.2% and the genetic difference between the French and the English is 0.1% for the RH negative trait. The genetic distance of several individual traits can then be averaged to compute an overall genetic distance.

Measures of Genetic Distance

There are several measures used to indicate genetic distance. These include:

Fixation Index

A commonly used measure of genetic distance is the fixation index which varies between 0 and 1. A value of 0 indicates that two populations are genetically identical whereas a value of 1 indicates that two populations are different species.

Nei's Standard Genetic Distance

This measure assumes that genetic differences arise due to mutations and genetic drift.

Cavalli-Sforza and Edwards 1967

This measure assumes that genetic differences arise due to genetic drift only.

Reynolds, Weir, and Cockerham's 1983

This measure assumes that genetic differences arise due to genetic drift only.

Noncoding DNA

In genetics, noncoding DNA describes components of an organism's DNA sequences that do not encode for protein sequences. In many eukaryotes, a large percentage of an organism's total genome size is noncoding DNA, although the amount of noncoding DNA, and the proportion of coding versus noncoding DNA varies greatly between species.

Much of this DNA has no known biological function and at one time was sometimes referred to as "Junk DNA". However, many types of noncoding DNA sequences do have known biological functions, including the transcriptional and translational regulation of protein-coding sequences. Other noncoding sequences have likely but as-yet undetermined function, an inference from high levels of homology and conservation seen in sequences that do not encode proteins but appear to be under heavy selective pressure.

Fraction of Noncoding Genomic DNA

The amount of total genomic DNA varies widely between organisms, and the proportion of coding and noncoding DNA within these genomes varies greatly as well. More than 98% of the human genome does not encode protein sequences, including most sequences within introns and most intergenic DNA.

While overall genome size, and by extension the amount of noncoding DNA, are correlated to organism complexity, there are many exceptions. For example, the genome of the unicellular *Polychaos dubium* (formerly known as *Amoeba dubia*) has been reported to contain more than 200 times the amount of DNA in humans. The pufferfish *Takifugu rubripes* genome is only about one eighth the size of the human genome, yet seems to have a comparable number of genes; approximately 90% of the *Takifugu* genome is noncoding DNA and most of the genome size difference appears to lie in the noncoding DNA. The extensive variation in nuclear genome size among eukaryotic species is known as the C-value enigma or C-value paradox.

About 80% of the nucleotide bases in the human genome may be transcribed, but transcription does not necessarily imply function.

Types of Noncoding DNA Sequences

Noncoding Functional RNA: Noncoding RNAs are functional RNA molecules that are not translated into protein. Examples of noncoding RNA include ribosomal RNA, transfer RNA, Piwi-interacting RNA and microRNA.

MicroRNAs are predicted to control the translational activity of approximately 30% of all protein-coding genes in mammals and may be vital components in the progression or treatment of various diseases including cancer, cardiovascular disease, and the immune system response to infection.

Cis-regulatory Elements

Cis-regulatory elements are sequences that control the transcription of a gene. Cis-elements may be located in 5' or 3' untranslated regions or within introns. Promoters facilitate the transcription of a particular gene and are typically upstream of the coding region.

Enhancer sequences may exert very distant effects on the transcription levels of genes.

Introns

Introns are non-coding sections of a gene, transcribed into the precursor mRNA sequence, but ultimately removed by RNA splicing during the processing to mature messenger RNA. Many introns appear to be mobile genetic elements.

Studies of group I introns from *Tetrahymena* indicate that some introns appear to be selfish genetic elements, neutral to the host because they remove themselves from flanking exons during RNA processing and do not produce an expression bias between alleles with and without the intron.

Some introns do appear to have significant biological function, possibly through ribozyme functionality that may regulate tRNA and rRNA activity as well as protein-coding gene expression, evident in hosts that have become dependent on such introns over long periods of time; for example, the *trnL-intron* is found in all green plants and appears to have been vertically inherited for several billions of years, including more than a billion years within chloroplasts and an additional 2–3 billion years prior in the cyanobacterial ancestors of chloroplasts.

Pseudogenes

Pseudogenes are DNA sequences, related to known genes, that have lost their protein-coding ability or are otherwise no longer expressed in the cell. Pseudogenes arise from retrotransposition or genomic duplication of functional genes, and become "genomic fossils" that are nonfuctional due to mutations that prevent the transcription of the gene, such as within the gene promoter region, or fatally alter the translation of the gene, such as premature stop codons or frameshifts. Pseudogenes resulting from the retrotransposition of an RNA intermediate are known as processed pseudogenes; pseudogenes that arise from the genomic remains of duplicated genes or residues of inactivated are nonprocessed pseudogenes.

While Dollo's Law suggests that the loss of function in pseudogenes is likely permanent, silenced genes may actually retain function for several million years and can be "reactivated" into protein-coding sequences and a substantial number of pseudogenes are actively transcribed. Because pseudogenes are presumed to evolve without evolutionary constraint, they can serve as a useful model of the type and frequencies various spontaneous genetic mutations.

Repeat Sequences, Transposons and Viral Elements

Transposons and retrotransposons are mobile genetic elements. Retrotransposon repeated sequences, which include long interspersed nuclear elements (LINEs) and short interspersed nuclear elements (SINEs), account for a large proportion of the genomic sequences in many species. Alu sequences, classified as a short interspersed nuclear element, are the most abundant mobile elements in the human genome. Some examples have been found of SINEs exerting transcriptional control of some protein-encoding genes.

Endogenous retrovirus sequences are the product of reverse transcription of retrovirus genomes into the genomes of germ cells. Mutation within these retro-transcribed sequences can inactivate the viral genome.

Over 8% of the human genome is made up of (mostly decayed) endogenous retrovirus sequences, as part of the over 42% fraction that is recognizably derived of retrotransposons, while another 3% can be identified to be the remains of DNA transposons. Much of the remaining half of the genome that is currently without an explained origin is expected to have found its origin in transposable elements that were active so long ago (> 200 million years) that random mutations have rendered them unrecognizable. Genome size variation in at least two kinds of plants is mostly the result of retrotransposon sequences.

Telomeres

Telomeres are regions of repetitive DNA at the end of a chromosome, which provide protection from chromosomal deterioration during DNA replication.

Functions of Noncoding DNA

Many noncoding DNA sequences have very important biological functions. Comparative genomics reveals that some regions of noncoding DNA are highly conserved, sometimes on time-scales representing hundreds of millions of years, implying that these noncoding regions are under strong evolutionary pressure and positive selection. For example, in the genomes of humans and mice, which diverged from a common ancestor 65–75 million years ago, protein-coding DNA sequences account for only about 20% of conserved DNA, with the remaining majority of conserved DNA represented in noncoding regions. Linkage mapping often identifies chromosomal regions associated with a disease with no evidence of functional coding variants of genes within the region, suggesting that disease-causing genetic variants lie in the noncoding DNA.

Some noncoding DNA sequences are genetic "switches" that do not encode proteins, but do regulate when and where genes are expressed. According to a comparative study of over 300 prokaryotic and over 30 eukaryotic genomes, eukaryotes appear to require a minimum amount of non-coding DNA. This minimum amount can be predicted using a growth model for regulatory genetic networks, implying that it is required for regulatory purposes. In humans the predicted minimum is about 5% of the total genome.

Some noncoding DNA sequences determine the expression levels of various genes. Other sequences of noncoding DNA determine where transcription factors attach. Some specific sequences of noncoding DNA may be features essential to chromosome structure, centromere function and homolog recognition in meiosis.

Noncoding DNA and Evolution

Shared sequences of apparently non-functional DNA are a major line of evidence for common descent.

Pseudogene sequences appear to accumulate mutations more rapidly than coding sequences due to a loss of selective pressure. This allows for the creation of mutant alleles that incorporate new functions that may be favoured by natural selection; thus, pseudogenes can serve as raw material for evolution and can be considered "protogenes".

Junk DNA

Junk DNA, a term that was introduced in 1972 by Susumu Ohno, was a provisional label for the portions of a genome sequence for which no discernible function had been identified. According to a 1980 review in *Nature* by Leslie Orgel and Francis Crick, junk DNA has "little specificity and conveys little or no selective advantage to the organism". The term is currently, however, an outdated concept, being used mainly in popular science and in a colloquial way in scientific publications, and may have slowed research into the biological functions of noncoding DNA. Several lines of evidence indicate that many "junk

DNA" sequences are likely to have unidentified functional activity, and other sequences may have had functions in the past.

Still, a significant amount of the sequence of the genomes of eukaryotic organisms currently appears to fall under no existing classification other than "junk". For example, one experiment removed 0.1% of the mouse genome with no detectable effect on the phenotype. This result suggests that the removed DNA was largely nonfunctional. In addition, these sequences are enriched for the heterochromatic histone modification H3K9me3.

Phylogenetic Footprinting

Phylogenetic footprinting is a technique used to identify transcription factor binding sites (TFBS) within a non-coding region of DNA of interest by comparing it to the orthologous sequence in different species. When this technique is used with a large number of closely related species, this is called phylogenetic shadowing.

Researchers have found that non-coding pieces of DNA contain binding sites for regulatory proteins that govern the spatiotemporal expression of genes. These transcription factor binding sites (TFBS), or regulatory motifs, have proven hard to identify, primarily because they are short in length, and can show sequence variation. The importance of understanding transcriptional regulation to many fields of biology has led researchers to develop strategies for predicting the presence of TFBS, many of which have led to publicly available databases. One such technique is Phylogenetic Footprinting.

Phylogenetic footprinting relies upon two major concepts:

1. The function and DNA binding preferences of transcription factors are well-conserved between diverse species.

2. Important non-coding DNA sequences that are essential for regulating gene expression will show differential selective pressure. A slower rate of change occurs in TFBS than in other, less critical, parts of the non-coding genome.

History

Phylogenetic footprinting was first used and published by Tagle et al. in 1988, which allowed researchers to predict evolutionary conserved cis-regulatory elements responsible for embryonic ε and γ globulin gene expression in primates.

Before phylogenetic footprinting, DNase footprinting was used, where protein would be bound to DNA transcription factor binding sites (TFBS) protecting it from DNase digestion.

One of the problems with this technique was the amount of time and labour it would take. Unlike DNase footprinting, phylogenetic footprinting relies on evolutionary constraints within the genome, with the "important" parts of the sequence being conserved among the different species.

Protocol

It is important when using this technique to decide which genome your sequence should be aligned to. More divergent species will have less sequence homology between orthologous genes. Therefore, the key is to pick species that are related enough to detect homology, but divergent enough to maximize non-alignment "noise". Step wise approach to Phylogenetic footprinting consists of :

1. One should decide on the gene of interest.
2. Carefully choose species with orthologous genes.
3. Decide on the length of the upstream or maybe downstream region to be looked at.
4. Align the sequences.
5. Look for conserved regions and analyse them.

Not all TFBS are Found

Not all transcription binding sites can be found using phylogenetic footprinting due to the statistical nature this technique. Here are several reasons why some TFBS are not found:

Species Specific Binding Sites

Some binding sites seem to have no significant matches in most other species. Therefore, detecting these sites by phylogenetic footprinting is likely impossible unless a large number of closely related species are available.

Very Short Binding Sites

Some binding sites show excellent conservation, but just in a shorter region than the ones we looked for. Such short motifs (e.g., GC-box) are often happened by chance in nonfunctional sequences and detecting these motifs would be challenging.

Less Specific Binding Factors

Some binding sites show some conservation but have had insertions or deletions. It is not obvious if these sequences with insertions or deletions are still functional.

Though they may still be functional if the finding factor is less specific (or less 'picky' if you will). Because deletions and insertions are rare in binding sites, considering insertions and deletions in the sequence would detect a few more true TFBSs, but it could likely include many more false positives.

Not Enough Data

Some motifs are quite well conserved, but they are statistically insignificant a specific dataset. The motif might have appeared in different species by chance. These motifs could be detected if sequences from more organisms are available. So this will be less of a problem in the future.

Compound Binding Regions

Some transcription factors bind as dimers. Therefore, their binding sites may consist of two conserved regions, separated by a few variable nucleotides. Because of the variable internal sequence, the motif cannot be detected. However, if we could use a program to search for motifs containing a variable sequence in the middle, without counting mutations, these motifs could be discovered.

Accuracy

It is important to keep in mind that not all conserved sequences are under selection pressure. To eliminate false positives statistical analysis must be performed that will show that the motifs reported have a mutation rate meaningfully less than that of the surrounding nonfunctional sequence.

Moreover, results could be more accurate if the prior knowledge about the sequence is considered. For example, some regulatory elements are repeated 15 times in a promoter region (e.g., some metallothionein promoters have up to 15 metal response elements (MREs)). Thus, to eliminate false motifs with inconsistent order across species, the orientation and order of regulatory elements in a promoter region should be the same in all species. This type of information could help us to identify regulatory elements that are not adequately conserved but occur in several copies in the input sequence.

Transcriptome

The transcriptome is the set of all RNA molecules, including mRNA, rRNA, tRNA, and other non-coding RNA produced in one or a population of cells. The term can be applied to the total set of transcripts in a given organism, or to the specific subset of transcripts present in a particular cell type. Unlike the genome, which is roughly fixed for a given cell line (excluding mutations), the transcriptome can vary with external environmental conditions.

Because it includes all *mRNA* transcripts in the cell, the transcriptome reflects the genes that are being actively expressed at any given time, with the exception of mRNA degradation phenomena such as transcriptional attenuation. The study of *transcriptomics*, also referred to as expression profiling, examines the expression level of mRNAs in a given cell population, often using high-throughput techniques based on DNA microarray technology. The use of next-generation sequencing technology to study the transcriptome at the nucleotide level is known as RNA-Seq.

Transcriptomics is the branch of molecular biology that deals with the study of messenger RNA molecules produced in an individual or population of a particular cell type.

Applications and Analysis

The transcriptomes of stem cells and cancer cells are of particular interest to researchers who seek to understand the processes of cellular differentiation and carcinogenesis. A number of organism-specific transcriptome databases have been constructed and annotated to aid in the identification of genes that are differentially expressed in distinct cell populations or subtypes; however, the analysis of relative mRNA expression levels can be complicated by the fact that relatively small changes in mRNA expression can produce large changes in the total amount of the corresponding protein present in the cell. One analysis method, known as Gene Set Enrichment Analysis, identifies coregulated gene networks rather than individual genes that are up- or down-regulated in different cell populations.

mRNA Regulation

Although microarray studies can reveal the relative amounts of different mRNAs in the cell, levels of mRNA are not directly proportional to the expression level of the proteins they code for. The number of protein molecules synthesized using a given mRNA molecule as a template is highly dependent on translation-initiation features of the mRNA sequence; in particular, the ability of the translation initiation sequence is a key determinant in the recruiting of ribosomes for protein translation. The complete protein complement of a cell or organism is known as the proteome.

A study of 158,807 mouse transcripts revealed that 4520 of these transcripts form antisense partners that are base pair complementary to the exons of genes. These results raise the possibility that significant numbers of "antisense RNA-coding genes" might participate in the regulation of the levels of expression of protein-coding mRNAs.

The Genographic Project

The Genographic Project, launched on April 13, 2005 by the National Geographic Society and IBM, is a multi-year genetic anthropology study that aims to map historical human migration patterns by collecting and analysing DNA samples from hundreds of thousands of people from around the world.

Overview

Field researchers at 11 regional centres around the world collect DNA samples from indigenous populations. The project also sells self-testing kits: for US$100 anyone in the world can order a kit with which a mouth scraping (buccal swab) is obtained, analysed and the DNA information placed on an Internet accessible database. The genetic markers on mitochondrial DNA (HVR1) and Y-chromosomes (12 microsatellite markers and haplogroup-defining SNPs) are used to trace the participant's distant ancestry, and each customer is provided with their genetic history. As of April 2010 more than 350,000 people had bought a test kit, and the success of the project has spawned a broader interest in direct-to-consumer genetic testing.

The Genographic Project is undertaking widespread consultation with indigenous groups from around the world. Genographic Project public participation kits are processed by Family Tree DNA (FTDNA) using the Arizona Research Labs at the University of Arizona.

The project is a privately-funded, not-for-profit collaboration between the National Geographic Society, IBM and the Waitt Family Foundation. Part of the proceeds from the sale of self-testing kits support the Genographic Project's ongoing DNA collection, but the majority are ploughed into a Legacy Fund to be spent on cultural preservation projects nominated by indigenous communities.

Team Members

Team members include:

- Spencer Wells, project director (National Geographic Explorer-in-Residence)
- Jin Li, principal investigator, East Asia
- Theodore Schurr, principal investigator, North America
- Fabricio Santos, principal investigator, South America
- Jaume Bertranpetit, David Comas and Lluis Quintana-Murci, principal investigators, Western Europe and Central Europe
- Pierre Zalloua, principal investigator, Middle East and Northern Africa
- Himla Soodyall, principal investigator, Sub-Saharan Africa
- Elena Balanovska, principal investigator, North Eurasia
- Ramasamy Pitchappan, principal investigator, India
- Alan Cooper, principal investigator, Ancient DNA
- John Mitchell, principal investigator, Australia and New Zealand
- Lisa Matisoo-Smith, principal investigator, Oceania
- Ajay Royyuru, head of computational biology, IBM
- Simon Longstaff, advisory board chair (director of the St James Ethics Centre)
- Meave Leakey, advisory board member
- Merritt Ruhlen, advisory board member
- Colin Renfrew, advisory board member
- Luigi Luca Cavalli-Sforza, advisory board member
- Wade Davis, advisory board member.

Use of Genetic Markers

The Genographic Project relies on the identification of genetic markers. Most human DNA is a shuffled combination of genetic material passed down the generations. There are, however, parts of the human genome that pass unshuffled from parent to child. These segments of DNA are only changed by occasional mutations—random spelling mistakes in the genetic code. When these spelling mistakes are passed down to succeeding generations, they become markers of descent.

Different populations have different genetic markers, and by following them through the generations scientists are able to identify the different branches of the human tree, all the way back to their common African root. Indigenous populations provide geographical and cultural context to the genetic markers in their DNA. These clues can help recreate past migration patterns.

Criticism

Shortly after the announcement of the project in April 2005, the Indigenous Peoples Council on Biocolonialism, (IPCB), released a statement protesting about the project, its connections with the HGDP, and called for a boycott of IBM, Gateway Computers, and National Geographic. Around May 2006, the United Nations Permanent Forum on Indigenous Issues (UNPFII) recommended suspending the project. Concerns were that the knowledge gleaned from the research could clash with long held beliefs leading to the destruction of their culture. They also feared that it could endanger land rights and other benefits.

In May 2006, the representatives of Indigenous went to UNPFII contesting any involvement in the testing. "The Genographic Project is exploitative and unethical because it will use Indigenous peoples as subjects of scientific curiosity in research that provides no benefit to Indigenous peoples, yet subjects them to significant risks. Researchers will take blood or other bodily tissue samples for their own use in order to further their own speculative theories of human history."

UNPFII conducted investigations into the objectives of the Genographic Project, and concluded that since the project was "conceived and has been initiated without appropriate consultation with or regard for the risks to its subjects, the Indigenous peoples, the Council for Responsible Genetics concludes that the Indigenous peoples' representatives are correct and that the Project should be immediately suspended.

As of December 2006 some federally recognized tribes in North America have declined to take part. "What the scientists are trying to prove is that we're the same as the Pilgrims except we came over several thousand years before," said Maurice Foxx, chairman of the

Massachusetts Commission on Indian Affairs and a member of the Mashpee Wampanoag. "Why should we give them that openly?" However, more than 50,000 indigenous participants from the Americas, Africa, Asia, Europe and Oceania had joined the project as of April 2010.

As of 2010, the consensus is that the Genographic Project's benefits of providing genetic knowledge to humanity have created stronger ties among various cultural groups. While indigenous rights groups' concerns have been addressed, other cultural interest groups likewise have asserted their rights. Various extended family organizations worldwide support the Genographic Project. They have found connections to their places of heritage. They have discovered kinship relations to other ethnic groups and nationalities, creating stronger and more peaceful ties with other polities. Participants have discovered their "roots," representing an inalienable right to cultural heritage.

Chapter 2

Postgenomic Chemistry

Deciphering the human genome will probably identify 5,000 to 10,000 new proteins of therapeutic relevance; some will be homologous to existing known targets, but many if not most will be entirely novel, with unknown structure and function.

Medicinal chemists know how to design and prepare molecules that can inhibit intracellular enzymes such as proteases, kinases, and phosphatases or modulate cell-surface or nuclear receptors with agonists or antagonists; indeed, many examples of such molecules have reached the drug market.

However, the arsenal of concepts, tools, technologies, and strategies that medicinal chemists use today are rather limited if the purpose is to control peptide-hormone/receptor interactions or protein-protein interactions.

Mimicking the interaction of hormones, such as follicle-stimulating or growth hormones, with their receptors or controlling cytokines signalling/transcription pathways are examples of such challenges we face at Serono International.

New tools must be invented and put in place beyond high-throughput screening (HTS) and peptide-phase display technologies. Such tools will be at the frontier of synthetic, medicinal, analytical, and computational chemistry; cheminformatics; HTS technologies; structural biology; and cell biology. Success will depend on how efficiently these areas cross-fertilize each other.

Thousands of new potential targets for drug discovery will be proposed by the genomics initiative. These numbers are huge compared with the pre-genomic era but are still very small when compared with the vastness of "chemical" space. Estimates of the number of possible "drug-type" small molecules—those with a molecular weight of less than 1,000—average around 1040. The largest pharma companies today have collections of discrete compounds that do not exceed 10 million.

In other words, the field of investigation for chemists remains essentially unexplored. Here, organic synthetic chemists will continue to play a major role by proposing new, original, sophisticated (3-D information-rich) yet readily accessible scaffolds or templates to be used in a combinatorial manner; inventing new reactions; developing new synthetic pathways; and extending their scope of application.

Such tools will be essential for medicinal chemists facing the post-genomic era. That's not all for chemists. One of the greatest challenges in the post-genomic era will be the validation of the most promising targets for therapeutic intervention.

Chemists can play a critical role by providing small molecules that alter gene function by selectively binding to their protein products. Having a small molecule partner for every gene product is the dream; such a molecule would then be evaluated in cell models and in vivo disease models, thus validating the protein target for drug discovery. This process is called "chemical genetics" and allows chemists to be involved in the drug discovery process before the target is validated; previously, medicinal chemistry programs started only after target validation.

Chemical genetics is based on constructive interactions between chemists and biologists; if successful, it will have spectacular advantages compared to the classical validation tools based on proteins mutants and knockout organisms. Chemical genetics offers conditional techniques and, more importantly, allows concurrent analysis of both the importance of a protein in a disease process (target validation) and a protein's amenability to functional modulation by a small molecule (target tractability). Having a small molecule partner for every gene product represents a fantastic opportunity to design the next generation of drugs in phase with the pharmacogenetics vision of the drug market, where drug responses are assessed on the basis of genetic disposition.

Besides new target identification, genomics will also lead to sharp diagnostic tools; it's expected that by 2025, everybody can have her or his genome sequenced. We will therefore move from the era of "disease"-specific compounds to the era of "disease and patient"-specific compounds in which drugs will be chosen on the basis of the phenotype/genotype of the diseased cell or tissue and the genome of the patient.

So the challenge for the future is to discover the right drug for the right patient at the right dose in the right time. Chemists will play a major role in this tough challenge, not only by providing new tools and concepts in their own field but also as essential members of multidisciplinary teams. This is particularly true in biotech companies like Serono where chemists find the research and innovation culture that will make it possible.

New Problems and Challenges

The past decade has been characterized by the dynamic integration of chemistry and biology. Chemistry as the science investigating structures and properties of molecules provides the fundamental basis for the development of biochemistry, molecular biology, and biotechnology. Chemical science actively investigates and employs the principles of molecular organization of biological processes in living systems.

Chemistry and chemical technology peculiarly use biological materials and catalysts to create steadily increased variety of useful molecules. Genomic research also has a great impact on related fields of modern science, including chemistry. The creation of a holistic system of knowledge of genetic nature, genetic materials, and structures of genomes has influence on the development of chemistry, providing it with evolutionary new representatives, methods, and molecular structures. In addition, the challenge of identification of chemical structure and function of all proteins in living organisms links chemical and biological science. The complete elucidation of the human genome and genomes of many other organisms is a remarkable scientific breakthrough that will affect our lives for decades to come.

The content of structural information generated as a result of genomics studies is huge. More than 500 genomes are already partially or completely sequenced. Genomes of various microorganisms, plants, animals, as well as the human genome, are among them. These studies allowed identification of 1.1 million nucleotide sequences that code for proteins.

However, there are certain limitations that need to be overcome before one can exploit successfully the wealth of information from genomic studies. Although not at the forefront during the past genomics efforts, chemistry will undeniably continue to play a crucial role in the biological sciences in the future. Therefore, one can predict a bright future for chemistry in the postgenomic era. For example, developments in physical, surface, and analytical chemistry will surely provide the basis of novel, improved detection methods that will speed up and facilitate diagnostics. Organic chemistry will influence biological sciences even more. Genomics provides chemistry with new possibilities, tasks, and challenges.

The functioning of a living organism is far more complex than the genome may suggest.

Therefore, profound studies of proteome, metabolome, cellome, and physiome are under way. Another important feature is the multidisciplinarity of problems, which can be solved only by the combined and concerted efforts of scientific teams, including experts from different disciplines (chemists, biologists, physicians, mathematicians, and others).

There is a need to discuss the directions of future developments in various fields of chemistry in view of and with respect to the developments in genomics. Obviously, the achievements of genomics and proteomics could considerably influence the classical chemistry as well as result in new scientific directions.

Identification of all Molecular Participants of Biological Processes

The fundamental and philosophical result of the genomic project is that all molecular representatives of the world of biological diversity can be identified.

Trace Element-containing Protein

Selenoproteins (SPs) are responsible for most biomedical effects of dietary applicable selenium and are important for mammals because selenium plays a significant role in many physiological processes, namely, in male reproduction, aging, immune function, and cancer prevention. The information about the human SPs potentially can be used for the further systematic clarification of mammalian SPs and their functions. It was established that SPs contain selenium in the form of selenocysteine (Sec), which was named as the 21st amino acid.

There are three terminating codones in the universal genetic code. It was discovered that one of them (UGA) has dual function, signalizing termination of protein synthesis as well as incorporation of such amino acid as Sec. Since then, classical methods of biochemistry and a variety of biophysical techniques are not enough to analyse the correct function of UGA. Most known selenoprotein genes have homologues, in which Sec is replaced with cysteine (Cys). Using that, specific approach was suggested for identification of SPs. It implies the search for the Sec/Cys-containing protein pairs of homologs.

In addition, to identify mammalian SPs, human and mouse (or human and rat) genomes were searched in parallel to identity pairs of Sec insertion sequence (SECIS) elements present in the selenoprotein genes. This method supported by the application of specially developed computer programs provided independent verification of a number of SPs in various genomes. Subsequent investigations of new SPs revealed examples of proteins with expression patterns limited to embryos or testes, as well as proteins with novel subcellular distributions. It was established that all characterized mammalian SPs are globular proteins. Sec is inserted into polypeptide chains during ribosome-based protein synthesis.

The expression of fusion SPs, containing a C-terminal green fluorescent protein (GFP) tag, and their following detection with antibodies to GFP by means of electron microscopy helped in revealing the first known plasma membrane SPs. It was found that the human genome has 25 selenoprotein genes and the mouse genome 24 ones. The further understanding of mechanisms of Sec insertion can assist in revealing approaches to the targeted insertion of this residue into proteins. These examples emphasize the power of bioinformatics in establishing of deep interrelation between genomics and chemistry.

Identification and characterization of new metal-containing proteins in humans and other organisms should set up new challenges and highlight the need for investigation of genomic and postgenomic chemistry of biological trace elements. Understanding of the identities and functions of trace elementcontaining proteins can also provide new tools for nonspecific incorporation of these elements into proteins.

Phosphotriesterases in all known Genomes

In recent years, of notable interest to us has been the study of triesterases, the enzymes catalysing hydrolysis of triesters of phosphoric acid. The enzymes of this class can accelerate the hydrolysis of a wide group of phosphoric acid derivatives including such supertoxic compounds as Sarin, Soman, Vx, many organophosphorus pesticides, and toxins. The enzymes of this class are applied as detectors of toxic organophosphates in biosensors and considered as major components in new protective systems against weapons of mass destruction.

We offered the mechanism of catalysis including the steps of the electrophilic activation of substrate reaction site by a complex with one metallic ion (CoI) in enzyme-active site and of the electrophilic activation of water molecule by a complex with a second metallic ion (CoII). The application of modern computer methods for comparison of sequence of nucleic acids coding protein synthesis allows the researchers to answer the question of existence of homologous proteins possessing phosphoesterase activity. Twenty-five proteins detected were highly homologous with the beststudied enzyme isolated from *Flafobacterium* sp. cells. The procedure for construction of the phylogenetic tree includes the combination sequences in clusters with the follow-up comparison of proteins by the principle of minimal deviations.

Structurally, the proteins unite in "branches"; the more similar the primary protein structures are, the closer they are located to one another on the phylogenetic tree. The necessary step in the active site formation and the catalytic activity manifestation is the presence of Lys169 in protein, the carbamylated form of which "collects" cobalt ions into a common active site and provides a necessary spatial closeness between substrate and water activation sites. It shows that, according to the presented data, human proteins and *E. coli* cells do not possess the organophosphate-related enzymatic activity.

Proteins of some microorganisms, such as *Mycobacterium*, *Sulfolobus*, *Mycoplasma*, and *Lystera*, show the potential enzymatic activity. This opens notable possibilities in search of new enzymes of this class.

Chemical Proteomics: Management of Biosystems by Selective Ligands

The regulation of many processes taking place in the biological systems can be organized through application of effectors special for some key biomolecules. Thousands of unknown proteins have been identified through genomic and proteomic research. It is important to discover specific molecules that can interact with them selectively to understand the role of newly discovered proteins and to regulate their activity. The main goal is to find one low-molecular-weight compound able to block or stimulate the activity of one protein in a highly selective way. This area can be identified as "chemical proteomics".

The goal of the chemical proteomics is the creation of "chemical keys" for all proteins existing in nature. Special interest to these tasks is dictated presumably by pharmacological importance.

More than 95 % of all human diseases are associated with defective gene expression or post-translation protein modification. Since that, specific molecular ligands can be very useful in explanation and restoration of the functions of biological macromolecules. They also can be used for construction of novel affinity tags to facilitate purification and detection of target proteins or polypeptides. The ligands helpful in control (suppression or activation) of gene expression have high importance.

Specific binding between proteins and their ligands is the molecular basis of all essential biological processes. The ways used in identification and characterization of protein sites interacting with other molecules are based on different strategies. One of the modern suggested ways is the following. Selection of appropriate site on the target protein, design of a complementary ligand compatible with the 3D structure of the site, construction of a limited solid-phase combinatorial library of near-neighbour ligands and solution synthesis of the hit ligand, immobilization, optimization, and application of the adsorbent for the purification of the target protein. This strategy is directed to the understanding of affinity and selectivity for enzyme inhibitors uses information from ligands and 3D structures of target proteins.

Combinatorial chemistry has emerged as a set of novel strategies for the synthesis of large sets of compounds (combinatorial libraries) for biological evaluation. Combinatorial approaches capable of generating libraries of different proteins allow the directed screening for a particular biological activity.

Analysis of proteins in complex with their ligands provides structural information on the amino acid residues involved in ligand binding. Synthetic chemistry enables one to create a large number of different molecules, including simple and more complex peptides, which may contain different amino acids, including unnatural ones, as well as non-peptide small molecules. The design and generation of synthetic molecules that can interfere with protein–ligand interactions represents a promising strategy for the explanation of protein structure and function. In addition to their basic significance, such synthetic proteomimetics are also useful tools for a range of biomedical applications.

A new very fast developing approach to the investigation of protein–ligand interactions is aimed at synthesis of molecules, which, owing to their specific molecular structure, are capable of mimicking the binding sites of natural proteins. Various protein-binding sites are composed of parts that are remote in the amino acid sequence, but brought into proximity by protein folding. They can be mimicked through scaffold peptides, in which the peptide fragments making up the binding site are presented through a molecular scaffold in a nonlinear, discontinuous fashion.

This task was initially accomplished by using short synthetic peptides to establish the linear binding sites of proteins. Such peptides, representing overlapping fragments of the protein, were tested individually for binding to the respective ligand in order to identify the protein region(s) responsible for the ligand recognition. The epitopes identified by this way were characterized and optimized regarding their binding affinity to the respective ligands.

Synthetic chemistry should play a significant role in the identification and functional characterization of gene products, as well as in the investigation of proteins' functions through controlled interference with the protein–ligand interactions.

Biocatalysis: Enzymes of New Generation

The methods of bioinformatics allow identification of comprehensive sets of genes encoding enzymes in various organisms as well as comparative and functional analysis of these proteins. For example, the problem of enzyme thermostability could be solved at the genetic level by comparing genomes of mesophilic and thermophilic microorganisms. Genomic access to thermostable enzymes and proteins may result in development of unique technologies of high-temperature biotechnological processes.

Enzymes are the most widespread catalysts that can be obtained from renewable raw materials.

Biocatalysis is the basis of important chemical processes. During the past two centuries, organic chemistry was substantially oriented toward the transformation of hydrocarbons and their different chemical derivatives, whereas the chemistry of the 21st century will be dealing with the problems of chemical transformation of renewable raw materials such as carbohydrates, biomass components, and carbon dioxide. Biocatalysts are the best tools for the chemical modification of molecules in the 21st century.

The detailed structural information at the atomic level is already known for a large variety of enzymes from X-ray crystallographic and NMR spectrometric methods. The existing concepts explain the observed effects of acceleration of chemical reactions and the nature of enzyme specificity and are based on fundamental physicochemical laws.

During the last 50 years, enzymes and biocatalytic systems were realized in the wide range of applications, including fine organic synthesis and multiple forms of chemical analysis. Enzymes provided the basis of many processes in food industry, industrial production, and utilization of detergents. They served as key components in environmental biotechnology and medicine and improved chemical and biological safety of various industrial processes.

Many "weaknesses" of enzymatic catalysis were overcome during the past decades. Thus, the methods of effective stabilization of enzymes were developed and the new conditions for their exploitation were discovered, and new methods of the use of enzymes in the media with organic solvents at increased temperatures were described. Methods of genetic engineering and site-directed mutagenesis played a significant role in elucidating reaction mechanisms of various enzymes and providing molecular basis for their biotechnological applications. Potentially all these features make enzymes the most effective biocatalysts. The up-to-date prognosis suggests that within one decade, total enzyme production in the world will reach the level of or even exceed the production of "classic" catalysts used in the chemical industry within the next decade.

The creation and construction of enzymes with new properties is based on the application of genetic information and modern achievements of genomics. It is possible to expect the appearance of new scientific directions of enzyme investigations and the development of new biocatalytical technologies.

The use of new methods of preparation of gene-expressed proteins obtained from unnatural amino acids might be capable of supporting the development of principally new catalysts, considerably widening the possibilities of biocatalysis. Biosynthesis of enzymes with unnatural amino acids included in the polymer chain could result in the development of new types of active sites, solving the problem of the use of enzymatic reactions under extreme conditions (extreme pH, temperature, salt content, etc.). The chemical modification of active sites by unnatural amino acids should result in the application of enzyme families with altered catalytic efficiencies and reaction mechanisms, and those that are characterized by transformed specificity and enantioselectivity.

In addition to methods traditionally used in protein design, such as DNA-shuffling, and directed evolution, it is anticipated that new methods allowing generation of enzymes with predefined properties will emerge. In this regard, the new methods allowing construction of proteins from the limited number of essential amino acids are quite attractive. These approaches should result in deeper understanding of physiological functions of proteins and lead to the appearance of new biocatalyst families of high applied significance.

Biocatalysis: New Resource Technologies

The limitations of traditional sources used in the chemical industry as well as limitations of hydrocarbon sources of energy, illustrate the need for development of new raw and energy sources. Growing interest in the biocatalytic conversion of biomass as the initial chemical raw materials for production of new materials, polymers, and energy sources (i.e., hydrogen, methane, ethanol, and diesel oil) may be envisioned as characteristic of the next decades. Significant progress may be expected in the development of biosystems catalysing the reduction of carbon dioxide to the basic carbon sources for the chemical industry (organic acids, alcohols, and monomers).

Enzyme Catalytic Sites and Mechanism of Catalysis from Sequence Data

Computer methods are widely employed in modern chemistry and molecular biology for various purposes. During the last decade, two approaches, bioinformatics and molecular modelling, have become especially popular and intensively developing areas. The methodology of bioinformatics is based on the informational analysis of nucleotide sequences and proteins. Within a framework of adequate physical considerations, molecular modelling allows to characterize protein structures and their changes induced by some treatments or local structural alterations. In combination with methods of molecular dynamics, molecular modelling represents a powerful approach that provides understanding of numerous physical and chemical aspects of protein molecules. Graphic capacities of modern work stations, relatively low cost and potency of modern processors, storage capacity of accumulated information, availability of a large number of resolved spatial protein structures, and nucleic acids and their complexes are the background for rapid worldwide distribution of computer modelling methods among scientists.

These methods of computer modelling are widely used for determination of structures of biological molecules (X-ray analysis and multimer nuclear magnetic resonance), theoretical studies of their interactions, studies of the interaction between membrane and membrane proteins, structural analysis of site-directed mutagenesis and prediction of new mutation sites, and protein structure prediction (method of homologous modelling).

Well-known software allow the construction of various biological molecules, edit their structure (by substituting some groups, changing conformation of molecular groups) followed by subsequent structural relaxation by means of methods of molecular mechanics and dynamics.

These programs also allow the calculation of various characteristics of the constructed molecules (e.g., electrostatic potential, solvent accessible surface, etc.), study of interactions between various molecules, alignment of protein sequences, creation of homology-based structures, and the investigation of ligand docking to active sites of enzymes.

Multiple Alignment of Amino Acid Sequences allows Recognition of the Enzyme Catalytic Site

Amino acid sequence determines structure and properties of each protein. Now, good evidence exists that in almost endless variability of proteins some structural elements are rather conservative, and these elements mainly determine the function of the protein molecule. This is especially demonstrative in the case of catalytic proteins. For example, in the case of hydrolases, which represent about one-third of all enzymes (about 1100 of 3700 enzymes) listed in the enzyme classification, only four main types of sites forming the catalytic structure are known. Consideration of active site structure of enzymes requires subdivision of the active site into two structural constituents:

- substrate-binding subsite, which is responsible for binding, fixation, and certain orientation of substrate(s); it determines enzyme specificity;
- catalytic subsite, which is responsible for chemical transformation of substrate molecule; this site usually employs general acid-base catalysis.

It is possible that within one large enzyme superfamily the substrate-binding subsite responsible for the enzyme specificity exists as quite variable protein structure corresponding to variations in the substrate structures. However, catalytic sites should represent rather conservative structural elements due to a limited number of catalytic site types. To test this hypothesis, we have employed the bioinformatic approach based on the comparison of amino acid sequences of proteins constituting one large family. We analysed results of sequence alignment of a few large enzyme families from HSSP database. These enzyme families were selected by the following criteria:

- the number of analysed enzymes should exceed 100; this provides reasonable statistical significance of the results;
- this analysis requires selection of enzymes with known active site structures and well documented catalytic mechanism.

One of the quantitative criteria of position conservatism for each residue in the protein sequence is the statistical criterion in the form of Shannon entropy. In information theory, Shannon entropy is one of the most important functions. The informational entropy (Shannon entropy) is a very convenient function for comparison of related proteins with distinct amino acid sequences.

The alignment procedure vs. some reference protein represents sequence positioning one over another one, followed by fixation of homologous sites, and recognition and eliminations of inserts. Such comparison of a large number of protein sequences allows the calculation of probability of localization of some amino acid residue in a certain position. This probability is determined as relative frequency of the amino acid j in a given position i.

Hydrolases were used as the object of research. Four mechanisms of water activation in reactions catalysed by these enzymes are known. They involve:

- aspartic (glutamic) acid carboxyl group, water activation by nucleophilic mechanism;

- histidine imidazole group, water activation by nucleophilic mechanism;
- complex with zinc or cobalt ions, water activation by electrophilic mechanism;
- complex with magnesium or manganese ions, water activation by electrophilic mechanism.

The following enzyme families representing these four mechanisms of water activation were chosen: pepsin family (activation by carboxyl group), chymotrypsin and subtilisin family (activation by imidazole group), alkaline phosphatase family (activation by complex with zinc or cobalt ions), pyrophosphatase family (activation by complex with magnesium or manganese ion).

Analysis of highly conservative amino acids (for which $Hj \sim 0$) revealed that during alignment, amino acid residues forming catalytically active subsites always represent conservative elements of the protein sequence. The catalytic site of acidic pepsin type proteases includes carboxyl groups of Asp31 and Asp215. These residues are recognized during alignment of amino acid sequences of pepsin family as conservative positions characterized by minimal value of Shannon entropy.

The catalytic site of the chymotrypsin family includes Ser195, His57, and Asp102, whereas the catalytic site of the alkaline phosphatase family includes Asp51, Asp369, His370, Asp327, His412, His331, and Ser102. Catalysis by inorganic phosphatase involves Glu20, Asp65, Asp70, and Asp102.

All these residues are recognized as conservative ones during multiple alignment of amino acid sequences of corresponding protein families. Thus, the bioinformatic approach allows recognition of side chains of amino acid residues forming a catalytic site of the enzymes and responsible for nucleophilic/electrophilic substrate conversion.

The comparison of enzyme amino acid sequences also revealed that Gly and Asp are the most frequently recognized as absolutely conservative residues. The finding that Gly is the most conservative residue was rather unexpected. Asp takes the second position in this list, and the sum of Gly and Asp represents about 50 % of all conservative residues recognized.

Amino acid residues were ranked by their conservatism in these four protein families.

For each amino acid, we determined its frequency as the conservative element ($Hj \sim 0$), normalization on total number of conservative positions for all amino acid residues in these families. Total frequency of conservative residues in enzymes completely differs from total frequency of amino acid residues in proteins, where Leu is the most frequent residues, whereas Gly takes only the fourth place in this list. (Frequency of Gly as the most conservative residue is 37 %.)

Gly, Asp, Cys, Pro, and His are the most frequent conservative residues in enzymes. They represent about 70 % of all conservative positions in these enzymes, whereas Met and Ile represent the most variable elements in the amino acid sequences. Thus, the most conservative residues can be separated into two principally different groups: (1) residues involved in substrate activation and acting as acids and bases (Asp and His); (2) residues forming active site architecture (Gly, Cys, Pro).

Aspartic Acid and Histidine in the Enzymatic Catalytic Cycle

The bioinformatic approach used in this study demonstrates a crucial role of aspartic acid and histidine residues in the functioning of the active site. Let us consider this role in more detail based on the analysis of mechanism of hydrolase action. As mentioned above, hydrolases represent the largest class of all known enzymes and their molecular mechanisms of catalysis have been well characterized. For most hydrolases, functional groups of amino acid residues constituting catalytic sites have also been identified and the interaction between these groups during catalytic cycle has been elucidated.

Based on the active site structure and mechanism of action all hydrolases can be arbitrary subdivided into the four main types:

- hydrolases containing aspartic or glutamic acid residues in the active site (lysozyme-pepsin type);
- hydrolases using imidazole group for water activation (the type of pancreatic ribonuclease, chymotrypsin, subtilisin, papain, lipase);
- hydrolases using complexes with Zn^{2+} or Co^{2+} for activation of water and substrate (type of alkaline phosphatase, carboxypeptidase A, and organophosphate hydrolase);
- hydrolases using Mg^{2+} and Mn^{2+} for activation of water and substrate (inorganic pyrophosphatase type).

Analysis of the catalytic mechanisms revealed that in most types of catalytic sites aspartic acid and histidine play principally important role.

Role of Gly in Formation and Conformational Flexibility of Active Structure

It is clear that conservative Gly residues do not play an important role in the activation of water molecules during the catalytic cycle because Gly does not have any substituent at the *alpha*-carbon atom, and therefore it lacks pronounced chemical function.

Nevertheless, Gly residues are essential for protein structure. This was demonstrated by mutation experiments where conservative Gly residues were substituted for any other amino acid. As a rule such substitutions resulted either in complete loss or significant decrease in catalytic activity. Apparently, conservative Gly residues are principally important for the following functions.

Being a unique amino acid with the most energetically favourable rotation along C–N and C–C bonds of polypeptide chain (Π and ψ Ramachandran angles) glycine may be a "junction point", providing change in the direction of polypeptide chain during "assembly" of amino acid residues into functionally competent active site. The essential role of Gly for structural function of enzyme-active sites was demonstrated by molecular modelling method. Thus, the presence of conservative glycines may explain the structural paradox of enzymatic catalysis, when completely identical active sites are formed from completely distinct protein sequences. They just share several common features such as the existence of conservative glycines and factors stabilizing the assembled structure. In this connection, we should mention that cysteine residues involved in disulfide bond formation (one of the most common stabilizing factors) take the third place in the rating of conservatism.

Conservative glycine residues may also function as a "hinge" responsible for known conformational flexibility of the active site. In many cases, conservative glycines are located near catalytically active residues. For example, the following conservative motifs were found in hydrolases from various families: Asp215XGly217 (pepsin), Asp170XXGly173 (thermolysin), Asp32XGly, His63Gly64, Gly119XSer221 (subtilisin), Gly17XSer177 (trypsin), His76Gly77, Ser153XGly155, Gly75XAsp177 (lipases). In these enzymes, Asp, Ser, and His residues are from the active site structures. For some enzymes, values of *phi* and *iota* angles for amino acid residues of the catalytic site are out of the energetically "relaxed limits". This was found for amino acid residues of *alpha*-chymotrypsin (His57, Asp102, Ser195) by using the Ramachandran map of these residues. The active site of these enzymes is conformationally tensed (values of Π and ψ angles are in an energetically unfavourable region).

In enzymatic catalysis, the conversion of initial substrate into reaction product(s) involves a series of intermediates possessing distinct structures. Conservative glycines of the active site may function as "relaxing" elements adapting active site conformation for the catalytic conversion of the next intermediate.

Cysteine and proline residues take top positions in the rating of amino acid conservatism. They are also essential for active site formation. Proline is a unique amino acid that unfolds the polypeptide chain.

Cysteine residues provide "required" active site structure by forming a disulfide bridge, which promotes fixation of catalytic residues (often located in different positions of a polypeptide chain) in the active site structure. For many enzymes, disulfide bond formation is the final step terminating active site assembly.

Enzymes vs. Classical Catalysts

A wide diversity of enzymes, great potentials of enzyme modification by genetic engineering methods, and a deep insight into enzyme-related mechanisms potentially provide their diverse applications. Enzymes are widely applied in fine organic synthesis, medicine, and analysis as active components of washing powders. Enzymes are most widely applied in the food industry.

However, enzymes can also be fairly competitive in solving some classical chemical tasks. As example, consider the problem of creation of catalysts for fuel cells. In view of progressing deficit of hydrocarbons, as a basis of modern power engineering, much attention is nowadays attracted to fuel cells, i.e., the electrochemical energy converters where fuel oxidation is spatially separated from reduction of oxidizer, usually air oxygen, resulting in the electrochemical potential generated on two electrodes. Fuel cells afford a direct conversion of oxidation energy to the electric form without the intermediate emission of heat. Due to this fact, the efficiency of fuel cells is fairly high, approaching

100 %. The electrocatalytic problem of fuel oxidation and oxygen reduction is quite involved. On the one hand, the electrocatalyst should accelerate the electron transfer from the electrode matrix to oxygen. On the other hand, it should take an electron out of the fuel molecule without intermediate formation of free-radical particles in both anodic and cathodic reactions. At present, hydrogen–oxygen fuel cells are most elaborated. Supposedly, the fuel cells are an alternative to the internal combustion engines for motorcars.

The only appropriate catalyst in catalytic and corrosive parameters for hydrogen–oxygen cells is metallic platinum. However, platinum, as electrocatalyst for fuel cells, has some principal drawbacks: first of all, the high price and sensitivity and, hence, the quantity of CO and H2S in the fuel.

CO actually totally and irreversibly inhibits platinum at 100 ppm concentration of the former in the fuel hydrogen. A principal limitation of platinum as catalysts in fuel cells for motorcars is imposed by highly limited resources for the world production of platinum. To-date, the world production is about 180 t platinum per year. To produce 60 million motorcars per year (the level of motorcar production in 2000), about 5800 t platinum are required according to the most modest estimates.

Biological catalysts are totally renewable and industrially producible in any necessary quantity.

To create the enzyme-based fuel cells, we applied hydrogenases (hydrogen oxidation enzymes) and blue copper-containing oxidases of laccase type (oxygen reduction enzyme). The fundamental ground for creation of enzyme fuel cells is the application of biocatalysis, i.e., the enzyme-catalysed acceleration of electrochemical reactions of electron transfer at the interface electronic conductor/ionic conductor upon direct "electric catalysis" between conductor and enzyme-active site.

The effect of direct electron transfer between conductor and enzyme-active site was disclosed in our laboratory and registered as the discovery (State registration No. 311, 1987). It should be noted that the USSR had the system of registration of priority research "discoveries", which did not follow from direct theoretical investigations, were unexpected, and promised novel technological advances. It was shown that at the electrodes made of any electron-conducting material, hydrogenase chemosorption in air oxygen establishes a reversible equilibrium of hydrogen potential.

At the electrodes with sorbed laccase, the potential is established that approached the equilibrium potential of oxygen reduction. Hydrogen and oxygen enzyme electrodes underlay the construction of the fuel cell, affording us to obtain a record coefficient of conversion for the free energy of hydrogen oxidation by oxygen, 95.7 %. The latest information on enzymatic hydrogen cells was presented elsewhere. The detailed comparison of electrochemical Behaviour of platinum and hydrogenase in hydrogen oxidation reaction showed that the exchange currents for hydrogenase by 2–3 factors higher than for platinum (referred to the catalyst active site). Note that the hydrogenase electrodes are not inhibited by H2S and practically not inhibited by CO.

Thus, for hydrogen activation reaction in electrochemical mode, it turned out that the enzymes have notably higher parameters than the "classical" catalyst. The possibility to produce enzymes in any necessary quantities is the ground for real practical creation of fuel cells with unique technological parameters as energy converters.

Chemically Modified Proteins: New Properties, New Capabilities

Structural and functional proteomics has already identified a large number of proteins with novel folds designed to carry out specific biochemical reactions. Some of these proteins have inspired chemists and biochemists to engineer artificial and semi-artificial proteins, which may be used in unprecedented industrial or pharmacological applications. Therefore, the preparation of "synthetic" proteins with improved properties can become a rapidly developing part of postgenomic chemistry.

Fluoro-containing Proteins and Organisms

The interest to the unnatural amino acid-containing proteins is stimulated by at least three aspects.

These are: (1) A potential possibility of the unnatural amino acid incorporation into proteins infinitely widens the spectrum of the novel proteins to be synthesized. The elaboration of the effective methods to synthesize the proteins and enzymes containing element-organic amino acid analogs gives us hope to obtain the proteins and enzymes with the properties previously unknown; (2) Novel classes of anticancer and antiviral agents could be proposed using the amino acid analogs and their derivatives; (3) The replacement of any amino acid significant part by their synthetic analogs is expected to lead to the formation of microorganisms with qualitatively novel properties. Amino-acyl tRNA synthetase is the key enzyme of amino acid recognition in the protein biosynthesis. Some analogs could not be incorporated into the proteins because of the high specificity of the above-mentioned synthetase.

Nevertheless, there are several main ways of unnatural amino acids' incorporation in protein structure. One way represents itself: cultivation amino acid auxotrophic *E. coli* strain with a cloned enzyme gene under the inducible promoter or in the presence of a specified protein expression inhibitor in a medium containing all natural amino acids. After significant biomass amount is accumulated, the medium is replaced and an amino acid analog is introduced in place of its natural counterpart. After a short incubation period, the protein expression is induced by the addition of inducer. The second way supposes chemical charging of the suppressor amino-acyl tRNA with the amino acid analog and an in vitro introduction of the analog at the nonsense mutated positions of the enzyme gene under investigation in the cell-free translation system. Another way to overcome the specificity of amino-acyl tRNA synthetase is mutagenesis of the enzyme. This approach may widen the enzyme specificity and enables one to incorporate the substances from a long analog list.

Realizing discussed approaches, the Tyr-auxotrophic strain *E. coli* B-2935 was transformed with plasmid pTES-His-OPH and inoculated in the medium containing F-Tyr. The biosynthesis of F-labelled organophosphate hydrolase was carried out. The mass-spectrometric analysis (MALDI-TOF) of purified protein testified to the replacement of 80 % Tyr-residues by their F-containing analogs (data not published).

It was shown that phenylalanine analog, namely, 4-fluorophenylalanine, can be introduced into the cellular protein by biosynthetic machinery. It was revealed that the relative content of FPA in the whole yeast protein from the cells grown up in the medium contained 1 mg/ml FPA.

Hybrid Proteins

The use of recombinant proteins has increased significantly in recent years as a response to the rapidly developed fields of proteomics. Recombinant hybrids containing a polypeptide fusion partner, termed affinity tag, to facilitate the purification of the target polypeptides are widely used. Many different proteins, domains, or peptides can be fused with the target protein. The production of recombinant proteins in a highly purified and well-characterized form has become a major task for the protein chemistry in the postgenomic era. Several different strategies have been developed to produce recombinant proteins on a large scale.

One approach is to use a very small peptide tag that should not interfere with the fused protein properties. The effect on tertiary structure and biological activity of fusion proteins with small tags depends on the location and on the amino acid composition of the tag. Another approach is to use large peptides or proteins as the fusion partner since the large partners can increase the stability and solubility of the target proteins. Some hybrid partners are specially used for the investigation of protein–protein interactions or changing properties of a target protein.

For example, the catalytic properties of organophosphate hydrolase containing oligohistidine sequence considerably differed from the native enzyme. The optimum pH for hybrid enzyme shifted to the basic area and became equal to 10.5 instead of 9.0 that was typical for the native enzyme. The thermostability of the developed enzyme increased, and temperature optimum of action shifted from 48 °C up to 55 °C. In addition to that, the effective constants for hydrolysis of many substances catalysed by the hybrid enzyme enhanced 10 times compared to the native form.

The wide application of green fluorescent protein as fusion partner opened new capabilities in the field of proteomics. The importance of affinity-tag technology will increase because of its necessity for the peptide/protein chip design, high-throughput purification, peptide/protein libraries, drug delivery systems, and strategies of large-scale production.

Postgenomic Macromolecular Chemistry

Future technology will be based on materials with excellent performance and novel functions. There is a large demand for so-called intelligent smart materials: self-recovery, self-adjustment or control, selfdiagnosis, stand-by capability for detecting nonlinear onset, ability to be externally tuned, etc.

Recombinant DNA technology can be utilized to produce polymers with specific properties and behavioural characteristics. The production of polymers by recombinant methods affords significant advantages over traditional polymer synthesis technologies, including control of microstructure, stereochemistry, and biocompatibility.

The production of artificial proteins by recombinant methods has already been demonstrated in several laboratories. Some groups have succeeded in the development of artificial proteins with smart properties. The electroactive polymers have been used to make artificial muscles. Hybrid intelligent hydrogels were developed via self-assembly of synthetic polymers and recombinant polypeptides.

Modern gene technology allows expression of any desirable amino acid sequence, and the recent breakthrough in industrial microbial cell fermentation and downstream processing of proteins allows production of large quantities of recombinant polymers. Precise control of the composition and structure of recombinant polymers renders them with unique properties. The introduction of unnatural amino acids in the structure of recombinant polymers will provide them with further unique properties not observed in natural polymers.

Recombinant polymers will combine both high mechanical and chemical stability as construction materials with the ability to react in a strong and predictable way to environmental changes and, hence, perform as active materials. In fact, these polymers will pave a way to soft machines where chemical energy is converted to mechanical energy with high efficiency utilizing the conformational transitions of polymers rather then movement of solid machinery.

The development and production of recombinant polymers is also a response to the demand for "green" alternatives to petroleum-based chemistry and waste-generating stoichiometric reagents. The recombinant polymers are produced by the environmentally friendly process of fermentation of microorganisms.

The resources needed for the production of recombinant polymers are renewable, and byproducts generated (e.g., microbial biomass) could be easily utilized and converted. Moreover, the recombinant polymers are biodegradable and pose minimal environmental threat as compared to traditional synthetic polymers.

One could easily foresee that recombinant polymers along with other natural polymers like carbohydrates, polyesters, and different composite materials based on these polymers, would to a large extent replace many traditional synthetic polymers.

Some of natural polymers are synthesized using template-guided synthesis. A classical example of this type of the synthesis is polymerase-catalysed replication of DNA molecules where novel chain is produced by one of two chains of primary DNA. In this case, it allows production of biomolecules identical to the template.

One could envision the development of this approach into several directions:

- development and investigation of chemical models of DNA polymerase; fine-tuning of conditions for the DNA proliferation in the systems in vitro with the use of chemical analogs of DNA copolymers;

- widening of possible application of enzymes (polymerases, oxidoreductases, esterases) for the template-directed matrix synthesis (polyaniline, polyethers, etc.); and

- investigation of catalytic synthesis of polymers that employ proliferation of polymer matrix; chemical models of polymerase chain reaction.

Investigations in this field should result in the creation of self-proliferating polymers. The new systems recording the information in chemical language different from the classical biological one could be suggested on the basis of a number of such polymers.

New Bioanalytical Chemistry

A number of new analytical technologies that qualitatively changed the face of modern bioanalysis have been developed in various genomic projects and their further applications. In addition to DNA sequencing methods, considerable progress was achieved in the development of biochip analytical devices and biosensors.

The development of proteomics illustrates the application of mass-spectrometry method for the analysis of proteins and peptides. Advances in genomics, in combination with the progress in nano/materials/info technologies, are being integrated to enable analytical devices and systems with potential global effects on individual and public health, safety, economic, social and political systems.

DNA microarrays have revolutionized the way of nucleic acid characterization. One can easily foresee that protein and small-molecule microarrays will have the same impact in many areas, such as protein structure–function and protein–protein interaction studies, as well as in lead compound identification. Toward such practical microarrays, novel chemistries that ensure selective, reliable, and efficient linkages of synthetic and biological molecules onto solid support are desperately needed. It is reasonable to believe that new reagents and chemoselective reactions operating in water will significantly improve the preparation of useful, stable microarrays that will find applications in many areas, especially in the drug development process.

General principles of DNA polymerase reactions and PCR technique initiated development of a number of atypical chemical processes. It was the first example of single-molecule registration.

A single enzyme molecule can generate polymerization and formation of nanoparticles that can play the roles of markers of immunological interactions and nucleic acid-based reactions. Scanning probe microscopy can be used as a counter of such nanoparticles. This approach promises to be extremely specific at registration of single molecular interactions.

Genome Projects of Micro-organisms

Biotechnology is a field of applied biology that involves the use of living organisms and bioprocesses in engineering, technology, medicine and other fields requiring bioproducts. Modern use similar term includes genetic engineering as well as cell- and tissue culture technologies.

The concept encompasses a wide range of procedures (and history) for modifying living organisms according to human purposes- going back to domestication of animals, cultivation of plants, and "improvements" to these through breeding programs that employ artificial selection and hybridization. By comparison to biotechnology, bioengineering is generally thought of as a related field with its emphasis more on higher systems approaches (not necessarily altering or using biological materials *directly*) for interfacing with and utilizing living things. The United Nations Convention on Biological Diversity defines biotechnology as:

> *"Any technological application that uses biological systems, living organisms, or derivatives thereof, to make or modify products or processes for specific use."*

Biotechnology draws on the pure biological sciences (genetics, microbiology, animal cell culture, molecular biology, biochemistry, embryology, cell biology) and in many instances is also dependent on knowledge and methods from outside the sphere of biology (chemical engineering, bioprocess engineering, information technology, biorobotics). Conversely, modern biological sciences (including even concepts such as molecular ecology) are intimately entwined and dependent on the methods developed through biotechnology and what is commonly thought of as the life sciences industry.

History

Biotechnology is not limited to medical/health applications (*unlike* Biomedical Engineering, which includes much biotechnology). Although not normally thought of as biotechnology, agriculture clearly fits the broad definition of *"using a biotechnological system to make products"* such that the cultivation of plants may be viewed as the earliest biotechnological enterprise. Agriculture has been theorized to have become the dominant way of producing food since the Neolithic Revolution. The processes and methods of agriculture have been refined by other mechanical and biological sciences since its inception.

Through early biotechnology, farmers were able to select the best suited crops, having the highest yields, to produce enough food to support a growing population. Other uses of biotechnology were required as the crops and fields became increasingly large and difficult to maintain. Specific organisms and organism by-products were used to fertilize, restore nitrogen, and control pests. Throughout the use of agriculture, farmers have inadvertently altered the genetics of their crops through introducing them to new environments and breeding them with other plants—one of the first forms of biotechnology. Cultures such as those in Mesopotamia, Egypt, and India developed the process of brewing beer.

It is still done by the same basic method of using malted grains (containing enzymes) to convert starch from grains into sugar and then adding specific yeasts to produce beer. In this process the carbohydrates in the grains were broken down into alcohols such as ethanol. Ancient Indians also used the juices of the plant Ephedra vulgaris and used to call it Soma. Later other cultures produced the process of Lactic acid fermentation which allowed the fermentation and preservation of other forms of food. Fermentation was also used in this time period to produce leavened bread. Although the process of fermentation was not fully understood until Pasteur's work in 1857, it is still the first use of biotechnology to convert a food source into another form.

For thousands of years, humans have used selective breeding to improve production of crops and livestock to use them for food. In selective breeding, organisms with desirable characteristics are mated to produce offspring with the same characteristics. For example, this technique was used with corn to produce the largest and sweetest crops.

In the early twentieth century scientists gained a greater understanding of microbiology and explored ways of manufacturing specific products. In 1917, Chaim Weizmann first used a pure microbiological culture in an industrial process, that of manufacturing corn starch using *Clostridium acetobutylicum,* to produce acetone, which the United Kingdom desperately needed to manufacture explosives during World War I.

Biotechnology has led to the development of antibiotics. In 1928, Alexander Fleming discovered the mold Penicillium. His work led to the purification of the antibiotic by Howard Florey, Ernst Boris Chain and Norman Heatley penicillin. In 1940, penicillin became available for medicinal use to treat bacterial infections in humans.

The field of modern biotechnology is thought to have largely begun on June 16, 1980, when the United States Supreme Court ruled that a genetically modified microorganism could be patented in the case of *Diamond v. Chakrabarty*. Indian-born Ananda Chakrabarty, working for General Electric, had developed a bacterium (derived from the *Pseudomonas* genus) capable of breaking down crude oil, which he proposed to use in treating oil spills.

Revenue in the industry is expected to grow by 12.9% in 2008. Another factor influencing the biotechnology sector's success is improved intellectual property rights legislation —and enforcement— worldwide, as well as strengthened demand for medical and pharmaceutical products to cope with an ageing, and ailing, U.S. population.

Rising demand for biofuels is expected to be good news for the biotechnology sector, with the Department of Energy estimating ethanol usage could reduce U.S. petroleum-derived fuel consumption by up to 30% by 2030. The biotechnology sector has allowed the U.S. farming industry to rapidly increase its supply of corn and soybeans—the main inputs into biofuels—by developing genetically modified seeds which are resistant to pests and drought. By boosting farm productivity, biotechnology plays a crucial role in ensuring that biofuel production targets are met.

Applications

Biotechnology has applications in four major industrial areas, including health care (medical), crop production and agriculture, non food (industrial) uses of crops and other products (e.g. biodegradable plastics, vegetable oil, biofuels), and environmental uses.

For example, one application of biotechnology is the directed use of organisms for the manufacture of organic products (examples include beer and milk products). Another example is using naturally present bacteria by the mining industry in bioleaching. Biotechnology is also used to recycle, treat waste, clean up sites contaminated by industrial activities (bioremediation), and also to produce biological weapons.

A series of derived terms have been coined to identify several branches of biotechnology, for example:

- Bioinformatics is an interdisciplinary field which addresses biological problems using computational techniques, and makes the rapid organization and analysis of biological data possible. The field may also be referred to as *computational biology*, and can be defined as, "conceptualizing biology in terms of molecules and then applying informatics techniques to understand and organize the information associated with these molecules, on a large scale." Bioinformatics plays a key role in various areas, such as functional genomics, structural genomics, and proteomics, and forms a key component in the biotechnology and pharmaceutical sector.
- Blue biotechnology is a term that has been used to describe the marine and aquatic applications of biotechnology, but its use is relatively rare.
- Green biotechnology is biotechnology applied to agricultural processes. An example would be the selection and domestication of plants via micropropagation. Another example is the designing of transgenic plants to grow under specific environments in the presence (or absence) of chemicals. One hope is that green biotechnology might produce more environmentally friendly solutions than traditional industrial

agriculture. An example of this is the engineering of a plant to express a pesticide, thereby ending the need of external application of pesticides. An example of this would be Bt corn. Whether or not green biotechnology products such as this are ultimately more environmentally friendly is a topic of considerable debate.

- Red biotechnology is applied to medical processes. Some examples are the designing of organisms to produce antibiotics, and the engineering of genetic cures through genetic manipulation.

- White biotechnology, also known as industrial biotechnology, is biotechnology applied to industrial processes. An example is the designing of an organism to produce a useful chemical. Another example is the using of enzymes as industrial catalysts to either produce valuable chemicals or destroy hazardous/polluting chemicals. White biotechnology tends to consume less in resources than traditional processes used to produce industrial goods. The investment and economic output of all of these types of applied biotechnologies is termed as bioeconomy.

Medicine

In medicine, modern biotechnology finds promising applications in such areas as

- drug production
- pharmacogenomics
- gene therapy
- genetic testing: techniques in molecular biology detect genetic diseases. To test the developing fetus for Down syndrome, Amniocentesis and chorionic villus sampling can be used.

Pharmacogenomics

Pharmacogenomics is the study of how the genetic inheritance of an individual affects his/her body's response to drugs. It is a coined word derived from the words "pharmacology" and "genomics". It is hence the study of the relationship between pharmaceuticals and genetics. The vision of pharmacogenomics is to be able to design and produce drugs that are adapted to each person's genetic makeup. Pharmacogenomics results in the following benefits:

1. Development of tailor-made medicines. Using pharmacogenomics, pharmaceutical companies can create drugs based on the proteins, enzymes and RNA molecules that are associated with specific genes and diseases. These tailor-made drugs promise not only to maximize therapeutic effects but also to decrease damage to nearby healthy cells.

2. More accurate methods of determining appropriate drug dosages. Knowing a patient's genetics will enable doctors to determine how well his/her body can process and metabolize a medicine. This will maximize the value of the medicine and decrease the likelihood of overdose.

3. Improvements in the drug discovery and approval process. The discovery of potential therapies will be made easier using genome targets. Genes have been associated with numerous diseases and disorders. With modern biotechnology, these genes can be used as targets for the development of effective new therapies, which could significantly shorten the drug discovery process.

4. Better vaccines. Safer vaccines can be designed and produced by organisms transformed by means of genetic engineering. These vaccines will elicit the immune response without the attendant risks of infection. They will be inexpensive, stable, easy to store, and capable of being engineered to carry several strains of pathogen at once.

Pharmaceutical Products

Most traditional pharmaceutical drugs are relatively simple molecules that have been found primarily through trial and error to treat the symptoms of a disease or illness.

Biopharmaceuticals are large biological molecules known as proteins and these usually target the underlying mechanisms and pathways of a malady (but not always, as is the case with using insulin to treat type 1 diabetes mellitus, as that treatment merely addresses the symptoms of the disease, not the underlying cause which is autoimmunity); it is a relatively young industry. They can deal with targets in humans that may not be accessible with traditional medicines. A patient typically is dosed with a small molecule *via* a tablet while a large molecule is typically injected.

Small molecules are manufactured by chemistry but larger molecules are created by living cells such as those found in the human body: for example, bacteria cells, yeast cells, animal or plant cells.

Modern biotechnology is often associated with the use of genetically altered microorganisms such as *E. coli* or yeast for the production of substances like synthetic insulin or antibiotics. It can also refer to transgenic animals or transgenic plants, such as Bt corn. Genetically altered mammalian cells, such as Chinese Hamster Ovary (CHO) cells, are also used to manufacture certain pharmaceuticals. Another promising new biotechnology application is the development of plant-made pharmaceuticals.

Biotechnology is also commonly associated with landmark breakthroughs in new medical therapies to treat hepatitis B, hepatitis C, cancers, arthritis, haemophilia, bone fractures, multiple sclerosis, and cardiovascular disorders. The biotechnology industry has also been instrumental in developing molecular diagnostic devices that can be used to define the target patient population for a given biopharmaceutical. Herceptin, for example, was the first drug approved for use with a matching diagnostic test and is used to treat breast cancer in women whose cancer cells express the protein HER2.

Modern biotechnology can be used to manufacture existing medicines relatively easily and cheaply. The first genetically engineered products were medicines designed to treat human diseases. To cite one example, in 1978 Genentech developed synthetic humanized insulin by joining its gene with a plasmid vector inserted into the bacterium *Escherichia coli*. Insulin, widely used for the treatment of diabetes, was previously extracted from the pancreas of abattoir animals (cattle and/or pigs).

The resulting genetically engineered bacterium enabled the production of vast quantities of synthetic human insulin at relatively low cost. According to a 2003 study undertaken by the International Diabetes Federation (IDF) on the access to and availability of insulin in its member countries, synthetic 'human' insulin is considerably more expensive in most countries where both synthetic 'human' and animal insulin are commercially available: e.g. within European countries the average price of synthetic 'human' insulin was twice as high as the price of pork insulin.

Yet in its position statement, the IDF writes that "there is no overwhelming evidence to prefer one species of insulin over another" and "[modern, highly purified] animal insulins remain a perfectly acceptable alternative.

Modern biotechnology has evolved, making it possible to produce more easily and relatively cheaply human growth hormone, clotting factors for hemophiliacs, fertility drugs, erythropoietin and other drugs. Most drugs today are based on about 500 molecular targets. Genomic knowledge of the genes involved in diseases, disease pathways, and drug-response sites are expected to lead to the discovery of thousands more new targets.

Genetic Testing

Genetic testing involves the direct examination of the DNA molecule itself. A scientist scans a patient's DNA sample for mutated sequences.

There are two major types of gene tests. In the first type, a researcher may design short pieces of DNA ("probes") whose sequences are complementary to the mutated sequences. These probes will seek their complement among the base pairs of an individual's genome. If the mutated sequence is present in the patient's genome, the probe will bind to it and flag the mutation. In the second type, a researcher may conduct the gene test by comparing the sequence of DNA bases in a patient's gene to disease in healthy individuals or their progeny.

Genetic testing is now used for:

- Carrier screening, or the identification of unaffected individuals who carry one copy of a gene for a disease that requires two copies for the disease to manifest;
- Confirmational diagnosis of symptomatic individuals;
- Determining sex;
- Forensic/identity testing;
- Newborn screening;
- Prenatal diagnostic screening;
- Presymptomatic testing for estimating the risk of developing adult-onset cancers;
- Presymptomatic testing for predicting adult-onset disorders.

Some genetic tests are already available, although most of them are used in developed countries. The tests currently available can detect mutations associated with rare genetic disorders like cystic fibrosis, sickle cell anemia, and Huntington's disease. Recently, tests have been developed to detect mutation for a handful of more complex conditions such as breast, ovarian, and colon cancers. However, gene tests may not detect every mutation associated with a particular condition because many are as yet undiscovered, and the ones they do detect may present different risks to different people and populations.

Controversial Questions

The absence of privacy and anti-discrimination legal protections in most countries can lead to discrimination in employment or insurance or other use of personal genetic information. This raises questions such as whether genetic privacy is different from medical privacy.

1. Reproductive issues. These include the use of genetic information in reproductive decision-making and the possibility of genetically altering reproductive cells that may be passed on to future generations. For example, germline therapy changes the genetic make-up of an individual's descendants. Thus, any error in technology or judgment may have far-reaching consequences (though the same can also happen through natural reproduction). Ethical issues like designed babies and human cloning have also given rise to controversies between and among scientists and bioethicists, especially in the light of past abuses with eugenics.

2. Clinical issues. These centre on the capabilities and limitations of doctors and other health-service providers, people identified with genetic conditions, and the general public in dealing with genetic information.

3. Effects on social institutions. Genetic tests reveal information about individuals and their families. Thus, test results can affect the dynamics within social institutions, particularly the family.

4. Conceptual and philosophical implications regarding human responsibility, free will vis-à-vis genetic determinism, and the concepts of health and disease.

Gene Therapy

Gene therapy may be used for treating, or even curing, genetic and acquired diseases like cancer and AIDS by using normal genes to supplement or replace defective genes or to bolster a normal function such as immunity. It can be used to target somatic (i.e., body) or gametes (i.e., egg and sperm) cells. In somatic gene therapy, the genome of the recipient is changed, but this change is not passed along to the next generation. In contrast, in germline gene therapy, the egg and sperm cells of the parents are changed for the purpose of passing on the changes to their offspring.

There are basically two ways of implementing a gene therapy treatment:

1. *Ex vivo*, which means "outside the body" – Cells from the patient's blood or bone marrow are removed and grown in the laboratory. They are then exposed to a virus carrying the desired gene. The virus enters the cells, and the desired gene becomes part of the DNA of the cells. The cells are allowed to grow in the laboratory before being returned to the patient by injection into a vein.

2. *In vivo*, which means "inside the body" – No cells are removed from the patient's body. Instead, vectors are used to deliver the desired gene to cells in the patient's body.

As of June 2001, more than 500 clinical gene-therapy trials involving about 3,500 patients have been identified worldwide. Around 78% of these are in the United States, with Europe having 18%. These trials focus on various types of cancer, although other multigenic diseases are being studied as well. Recently, two children born with severe combined immunodeficiency disorder ("SCID") were reported to have been cured after being given genetically engineered cells. Gene therapy faces many obstacles before it can become a practical approach for treating disease. At least four of these obstacles are as follows:

1. *Gene delivery tools.* Genes are inserted into the body using gene carriers called vectors. The most common vectors now are viruses, which have evolved a way of encapsulating and delivering their genes to human cells in a pathogenic manner. Scientists manipulate the genome of the virus by removing the disease-causing genes and inserting the therapeutic genes. However, while viruses are effective, they can introduce problems like toxicity, immune and inflammatory responses, and gene control and targeting issues. In addition, in order for gene therapy to provide permanent therapeutic effects, the

introduced gene needs to be integrated within the host cell's genome. Some viral vectors effect this in a random fashion, which can introduce other problems such as disruption of an endogenous host gene.

2. *High costs.* Since gene therapy is relatively new and at an experimental stage, it is an expensive treatment to undertake. This explains why current studies are focused on illnesses commonly found in developed countries, where more people can afford to pay for treatment. It may take decades before developing countries can take advantage of this technology.

3. *Limited knowledge of the functions of genes.* Scientists currently know the functions of only a few genes. Hence, gene therapy can address only some genes that cause a particular disease. Worse, it is not known exactly whether genes have more than one function, which creates uncertainty as to whether replacing such genes is indeed desirable.

4. *Multigene disorders and effect of environment.* Most genetic disorders involve more than one gene. Moreover, most diseases involve the interaction of several genes and the environment. For example, many people with cancer not only inherit the disease gene for the disorder, but may have also failed to inherit specific tumour suppressor genes. Diet, exercise, smoking and other environmental factors may have also contributed to their disease.

Human Genome Project

The Human Genome Project is an initiative of the U.S. Department of Energy ("DOE") that aims to generate a high-quality reference sequence for the entire human genome and identify all the human genes.

The DOE and its predecessor agencies were assigned by the U.S. Congress to develop new energy resources and technologies and to pursue a deeper understanding of potential health and environmental risks posed by their production and use. In 1986, the DOE announced its Human Genome Initiative. Shortly thereafter, the DOE and National Institutes of Health developed a plan for a joint Human Genome Project ("HGP"), which officially began in 1990.

The HGP was originally planned to last 15 years. However, rapid technological advances and worldwide participation accelerated the completion date to 2003 (making it a 13 year project). Already it has enabled gene hunters to pinpoint genes associated with more than 30 disorders.

Cloning

Cloning involves the removal of the nucleus from one cell and its placement in an unfertilized egg cell whose nucleus has either been deactivated or removed.

There are two types of cloning:

1. Reproductive cloning. After a few divisions, the egg cell is placed into a uterus where it is allowed to develop into a fetus that is genetically identical to the donor of the original nucleus.

2. Therapeutic cloning. The egg is placed into a Petri dish where it develops into embryonic stem cells, which have shown potentials for treating several ailments.

In February 1997, cloning became the focus of media attention when Ian Wilmut and his colleagues at the Roslin Institute announced the successful cloning of a sheep, named Dolly, from the mammary glands of an adult female. The cloning of Dolly made it apparent to many that the techniques used to produce her could someday be used to clone human beings. This stirred a lot of controversy because of its ethical implications.

Agriculture

Crop Yield: Using the techniques of modern biotechnology, one or two genes (Smartstax from Monsanto in collaboration with Dow AgroSciences will use 8, starting in 2010) may be transferred to a highly developed crop variety to impart a new character that would increase its yield. However, while increases in crop yield are the most obvious applications of modern biotechnology in agriculture, it is also the most difficult one. Current genetic engineering techniques work best for effects that are controlled by a single gene. Many of the genetic characteristics associated with yield (e.g., enhanced growth) are controlled by a large number of genes, each of which has a minimal effect on the overall yield. There is, therefore, much scientific work to be done in this area.

Reduced Vulnerability of Crops to Environmental Stresses

Crops containing genes that will enable them to withstand biotic and abiotic stresses may be developed. For example, drought and excessively salty soil are two important limiting factors in crop productivity. Biotechnologists are studying plants that can cope with these extreme conditions in the hope of finding the genes that enable them to do so and eventually transferring these genes to the more desirable crops. One of the latest developments is the identification of a plant gene, At-DBF2, from Arabidopsis thaliana, a tiny weed that is often used for plant research because it is very easy to grow and its genetic code is well mapped out. When this gene was inserted into tomato and tobacco cells, the cells were able to withstand environmental stresses like salt, drought, cold and heat, far more than ordinary cells. If these preliminary results prove successful in larger trials, then At-DBF2 genes can help in engineering crops that can better withstand harsh environments. Researchers have also created transgenic rice plants that are resistant to rice yellow mottle virus (RYMV). In Africa, this virus destroys majority of the rice crops and makes the surviving plants more susceptible to fungal infections.

Increased Nutritional Qualities

Proteins in foods may be modified to increase their nutritional qualities. Proteins in legumes and cereals may be transformed to provide the amino acids needed by human beings for a balanced diet. A good example is the work of Professors Ingo Potrykus and Peter Beyer in creating Golden rice (discussed below).

Improved Taste, Texture or Appearance of Food

Modern biotechnology can be used to slow down the process of spoilage so that fruit can ripen longer on the plant and then be transported to the consumer with a still reasonable shelf life. This alters the taste, texture and appearance of the fruit. More importantly, it could expand the market for farmers in developing countries due to the reduction in spoilage. However, there is sometimes a lack of understanding by researchers in developed countries about the actual needs of prospective beneficiaries in developing countries. For example, engineering soybeans to resist spoilage makes them less suitable for producing tempeh which is a significant source of protein that depends on fermentation. The use of modified soybeans results in a lumpy texture that is less palatable and less convenient when cooking.

The first genetically modified food product was a tomato which was transformed to delay its ripening. Researchers in Indonesia, Malaysia, Thailand, Philippines and Vietnam are currently working on delayed-ripening papaya in collaboration with the University of Nottingham and Zeneca.

Biotechnology in cheese production: enzymes produced by micro-organisms provide an alternative to animal rennet – a cheese coagulant – and an alternative supply for cheese makers. This also eliminates possible public concerns with animal-derived material, although there are currently no plans to develop synthetic milk, thus making this argument less compelling. Enzymes offer an animal-friendly alternative to animal rennet. While providing comparable quality, they are theoretically also less expensive.

About 85 million tons of wheat flour is used every year to bake bread. By adding an enzyme called maltogenic amylase to the flour, bread stays fresher longer. Assuming that 10–15% of bread is thrown away as stale, if it could be made to stay fresh another 5–7 days then perhaps 2 million tons of flour per year would be saved. Other enzymes can cause bread to expand to make a lighter loaf, or alter the loaf in a range of ways.

Reduced Dependence on Fertilizers, Pesticides and other Agrochemicals

Most of the current commercial applications of modern biotechnology in agriculture are on reducing the dependence of farmers on agrochemicals. For example, *Bacillus thuringiensis* (Bt) is a soil bacterium that produces a protein with insecticidal qualities. Traditionally, a fermentation process has been used to produce an insecticidal spray from these bacteria. In this form, the Bt toxin occurs as an inactive protoxin, which requires digestion by an insect to be effective.

There are several Bt toxins and each one is specific to certain target insects. Crop plants have now been engineered to contain and express the genes for Bt toxin, which they produce in its active form. When a susceptible insect ingests the transgenic crop cultivar expressing the Bt protein, it stops feeding and soon thereafter dies as a result of the Bt toxin binding to its gut wall. Bt corn is now commercially available in a number of countries to control corn borer (a lepidopteran insect), which is otherwise controlled by spraying (a more difficult process).

Crops have also been genetically engineered to acquire tolerance to broad-spectrum herbicide. The lack of herbicides with broad-spectrum activity and no crop injury was a consistent limitation in crop weed management. Multiple applications of numerous herbicides were routinely used to control a wide range of weed species detrimental to agronomic crops. Weed management tended to rely on preemergence—that is, herbicide applications were sprayed in response to expected weed infestations rather than in response to actual weeds present. Mechanical cultivation and hand weeding were often necessary to control weeds not controlled by herbicide applications.

The introduction of herbicide-tolerant crops has the potential of reducing the number of herbicide active ingredients used for weed management, reducing the number of herbicide applications made during a season, and increasing yield due to improved weed management and less crop injury. Transgenic crops that express tolerance to glyphosate, glufosinate and bromoxynil have been developed. These herbicides can now be sprayed on transgenic crops without inflicting damage on the crops while killing nearby weeds.

From 1996 to 2001, herbicide tolerance was the most dominant trait introduced to commercially available transgenic crops, followed by insect resistance. In 2001, herbicide tolerance deployed in soybean, corn and cotton accounted for 77% of the 626,000 square kilometres planted to transgenic crops; Bt crops accounted for 15%; and "stacked genes" for herbicide tolerance and insect resistance used in both cotton and corn accounted for 8%.

Production of Novel Substances in Crop Plants

Biotechnology is being applied for novel uses other than food. For example, oilseed can be modified to produce fatty acids for detergents, substitute fuels and petrochemicals. Potatoes, tomatoes, rice tobacco, lettuce, safflowers, and other plants have been genetically engineered to produce insulin and certain vaccines. If future clinical trials prove successful, the advantages of edible vaccines would be enormous, especially for developing countries.

The transgenic plants may be grown locally and cheaply. Homegrown vaccines would also avoid logistical and economic problems posed by having to transport traditional preparations over long distances and keeping them cold while in transit. And since they are edible, they will not need syringes, which are not only an additional expense in the traditional vaccine preparations but also a source of infections if contaminated.

In the case of insulin grown in transgenic plants, it is well-established that the gastrointestinal system breaks the protein down therefore this could not currently be administered as an edible protein. However, it might be produced at significantly lower cost than insulin produced in costly bioreactors. For example, Calgary, Canada-based SemBioSys Genetics, Inc. reports that its safflower-produced insulin will reduce unit costs by over 25% or more and approximates a reduction in the capital costs associated with building a commercial-scale insulin manufacturing facility of over $100 million, compared to traditional biomanufacturing facilities.

Criticism

There is another side to the agricultural biotechnology issue. It includes increased herbicide usage and resultant herbicide resistance, "super weeds," residues on and in food crops, genetic contamination of non-GM crops which hurt organic and conventional farmers, etc.

Biological Engineering

Biotechnological engineering or biological engineering is a branch of engineering that focuses on biotechnologies and biological science. It includes different disciplines such as biochemical engineering, biomedical engineering, bio-process engineering, biosystem engineering and so on. Because of the novelty of the field, the definition of a bioengineer is still undefined. However, in general it is an integrated approach of fundamental biological sciences and traditional engineering principles. Biotechnologists are often employed to scale up bio processes from the laboratory scale to the manufacturing scale. Moreover, as with most engineers, they often deal with management, economic and legal issues. Since patents and regulation (e.g., U.S. Food and Drug Administration regulation in the U.S.) are very important issues for biotech enterprises, bioengineers are often required to have knowledge related to these issues.

The increasing number of biotech enterprises is likely to create a need for bioengineers in the years to come. Many universities throughout the world are now providing programs in bioengineering and biotechnology (as independent programs or specialty programs within more established engineering fields).

Bioremediation and Biodegradation

Biotechnology is being used to engineer and adapt organisms especially microorganisms in an effort to find sustainable ways to clean up contaminated environments. The elimination of a wide range of pollutants and wastes from the environment is an absolute requirement to promote a sustainable development of our society with low environmental impact.

Biological processes play a major role in the removal of contaminants and biotechnology is taking advantage of the astonishing catabolic versatility of microorganisms to degrade/convert such compounds. New methodological breakthroughs in sequencing, genomics, proteomics, bioinformatics and imaging are producing vast amounts of information.

In the field of Environmental Microbiology, genome-based global studies open a new era providing unprecedented *in silico* views of metabolic and regulatory networks, as well as clues to the evolution of degradation pathways and to the molecular adaptation strategies to changing environmental conditions. Functional genomic and metagenomic approaches are increasing our understanding of the relative importance of different pathways and regulatory networks to carbon flux in particular environments and for particular compounds and they will certainly accelerate the development of bioremediation technologies and biotransformation processes.

Marine environments are especially vulnerable since oil spills of coastal regions and the open sea are poorly containable and mitigation is difficult. In addition to pollution through human activities, millions of tons of petroleum enter the marine environment every year from natural seepages. Despite its toxicity, a considerable fraction of petroleum oil entering marine systems is eliminated by the hydrocarbon-degrading activities of microbial communities, in particular by a remarkable recently discovered group of specialists, the so-called hydrocarbonoclastic bacteria (HCCB).

Biotechnology Regulations

The National Institute of Health was the first federal agency to assume regulatory responsibility in the United States. The Recombinant DNA Advisory Committee of the NIH published guidelines for working with recombinant DNA and recombinant organisms in the laboratory. Nowadays, the agencies that are responsible for the biotechnology regulation are: US Department of Agriculture (USDA) that regulates plant pests and medical preparation from living organisms, Environmental Protection Agency (EPA) that regulates pesticides and herbicides, and the Food and Drug Administration (FDA) which ensures that the food and drug products are safe and effective

The Next Human Genome Project: Our Microbes

A proposed project to sequence the microorganisms that inhabit our bodies could have a huge impact on human health.

Much as we might like to ignore them, microbes have colonized almost every inch of our bodies, living in our mouths, skin, lungs, and gut. Indeed, the human body has 10 times as many microbial cells as human cells. They're a vital part of our health, breaking down otherwise indigestible foods, making essential vitamins, and even shaping our immune system. Recent research suggests that microbes play a role in diseases, such as ulcers, heart disease, and obesity.

While microbes make up such an intimate part of us, most of our microbial inhabitants remain a mystery. The bacteria in the human body are very difficult to study, since only about 1 percent of them can be grown in the lab. Now a proposed new project to sequence all our microbial residents could change that

> "This is completely unexplored territory that is likely to have a large impact on our understanding of human health and disease," says George Weinstock, codirector of the Human Sequencing Centre at the Baylor College of Medicine, in Houston. "We hadn't been able to approach it because of the scale of the problem. But now we are finally able to open that door."

Thanks to ever-improving methods to sequence DNA, scientists can now analyse the genomes of entire microbial communities, a field known as metagenomics. By comparing microbial communities in people of different ages, origins, and health statuses, researchers hope to find out precisely how microorganisms prevent or increase risk for certain diseases and whether they can be manipulated to improve health.

Several metagenomics projects are under way or have been completed, including analysis of the microbes living in the human gut and on the skin. But a true snapshot of our microbial menagerie will require a massive effort, along the lines of the Human Genome Project. "Even though a microbial genome is one-thousandth the size of the human genome, the total number of microbial genes in [the human] body is much greater than human genes because you have so many different species," says Weinstock. The National Institutes of Health (NIH) is now considering such a project. Metagenomics experts and government officials met last week to determine if the proposal, dubbed the human microbiome, will become an NIH "Roadmap" initiative. These NIH-wide programs identify major gaps in biomedical research and provide financial support on a much larger scale than typical grants.

Recent research from Gordon's lab hints at the potential public-health impact of a clearer understanding of our microbial tenants. Gordon and his colleagues have shown that obese people harbor different microbial communities than lean people. And as obese people lost weight, their microbes began to look more like their lean counterparts' microbes. Researchers aren't yet sure what triggers the differences, but they found in a similar study in mice that the microbial populations of obese mice could more effectively release calories from food during digestion than could microbes of their lean littermates.

While exciting, Gordon's research also illustrates the challenges of cataloguing microbes. To truly interpret the human microbiome, scientists will need to look at the variation in microbial communities among many people and a variety of populations. Complicating the problem is that, while an individual's human genome is static, a person's microbial composition—and thus his or her microbiome—fluctuates over time. So an accurate picture of one person's microbiome could require multiple resequencing efforts.

These types of studies could yield the biggest reward, revealing whether different organisms are correlated with different health states. Gordon and others hope that a microbial analysis will ultimately become a routine part of medical exams, perhaps used to diagnose different diseases.

Scientists are still debating whether the microbiome will become a road-map project, and if so, what the final goals of the project will be: should they focus on generating complete sequences of dominant microbes, for example, or devote equal energy to the complex task of studying microbial variation?

Inborn Error of Metabolism

Inborn errors of metabolism comprise a large class of genetic diseases involving disorders of metabolism. The majority are due to defects of single genes that code for enzymes that facilitate conversion of various substances (substrates) into others (products). In most of the disorders, problems arise due to accumulation of substances which are toxic or interfere with normal function, or to the effects of reduced ability to synthesize essential compounds. Inborn errors of metabolism are now often referred to as congenital metabolic diseases or inherited metabolic diseases.

The term *inborn error of metabolism* was coined by a British physician, Archibald Garrod (1857–1936), in the early 20th century (1908). He is known for work that prefigured the "one gene-one enzyme" hypothesis, based on his studies on the nature and inheritance of alkaptonuria. His seminal text, *Inborn Errors of Metabolism* was published in 1923.

Major Categories of Inherited Metabolic Diseases

Traditionally the inherited metabolic diseases were categorized as disorders of carbohydrate metabolism, amino acid metabolism, organic acid metabolism, or lysosomal storage diseases. In recent decades, hundreds of new inherited disorders of metabolism have been discovered and the categories have proliferated. Following are some of the major classes of congenital metabolic diseases, with prominent examples of each class. Many others do not fall into these categories. ICD-10 codes are provided where available.

- Disorders of carbohydrate metabolism
    - E.g., glycogen storage disease
- Disorders of amino acid metabolism
    - E.g., phenylketonuria, maple syrup urine disease, glutaric acidemia type 1
- Disorders of organic acid metabolism (organic acidurias)
    - E.g., alcaptonuria
- Disorders of fatty acid oxidation and mitochondrial metabolism
    - E.g., medium chain acyl dehydrogenase deficiency (glutaric acidemia type 2)
- Disorders of porphyrin metabolism
    - E.g., acute intermittent porphyria
- Disorders of purine or pyrimidine metabolism
    - E.g., Lesch-Nyhan syndrome

- Disorders of steroid metabolism
  - E.g., congenital adrenal hyperplasia
- Disorders of mitochondrial function
  - E.g., Kearns-Sayre syndrome
- Disorders of peroxisomal function
  - E.g., Zellweger syndrome
- Lysosomal storage disorders
  - E.g., Gaucher's disease
  - E.g., Niemann Pick disease.

Incidence

In a study in British Columbia, the overall incidence of the inborn errors of metabolism were estimated to be 70 per 100,000 live births or 1 in 1,400 births, overall representing more than approximately 15% of single gene disorders in the population.

Manifestations and Presentations

Because of the enormous number of these diseases and wide range of systems affected, nearly every "presenting complaint" to a doctor may have a congenital metabolic disease as a possible cause, especially in childhood. The following are examples of potential manifestations affecting each of the major organ systems:

- Growth failure, failure to thrive, weight loss
- Ambiguous genitalia, delayed puberty, precocious puberty
- Developmental delay, seizures, dementia, encephalopathy, stroke
- Deafness, blindness, pain agnosia
- Skin rash, abnormal pigmentation, lack of pigmentation, excessive hair growth, lumps and bumps
- Dental abnormalities
- Immunodeficiency, thrombocytopenia, anemia, enlarged spleen, enlarged lymph nodes
- Many forms of cancer
- Recurrent vomiting, diarrhea, abdominal pain
- Excessive urination, renal failure, dehydration, edema
- Hypotension, heart failure, enlarged heart, hypertension, myocardial infarction

- Hepatomegaly, jaundice, liver failure
- Unusual facial features, congenital malformations
- Excessive breathing (hyperventilation), respiratory failure
- Abnormal Behaviour, depression, psychosis
- Joint pain, muscle weakness, cramps
- Hypothyroidism, adrenal insufficiency, hypogonadism, diabetes mellitus.

Diagnostic Techniques

Dozens of congenital metabolic diseases are now detectable by newborn screening tests, especially the expanded testing using mass spectrometry. This is an increasingly common way for the diagnosis to be made and sometimes results in earlier treatment and a better outcome. There is a revolutionary GC/MS based technology with an integrated analytics system, which has now made it possible to test a newborn for over 100 genetic metabolic disorders.

Because of the multiplicity of conditions, many different diagnostic tests are used for screening. An abnormal result is often followed by a subsequent "definitive test" to confirm the suspected diagnosis.

Common screening tests used in the last sixty years:

- Ferric chloride test (turned colours in reaction to various abnormal metabolites in urine)
- Ninhydrin paper chromatography (detected abnormal amino acid patterns)
- Guthrie bacterial inhibition assay (detected a few amino acids in excessive amounts in blood) The dried blood spot can be used for multianalyte testing using Tandem Mass Spectroscopy (MS/MS). This given an indication for a disorder. The same has to be further confirmed by enzyme assays, GC/MS or DNA Testing.
- Quantitative measurement of amino acids in plasma and urine
- Urine organic acid analysis by Gas chromatography-mass spectrometry
- Plasma acylcarnitines analysis by mass spectrometry
- Urine purines and pyrimidines analysis by Gas chromatography-mass spectrometry.

Specific diagnostic tests (or focused screening for a small set of disorders):

- Tissue biopsy or necropsy: liver, muscle, brain, bone marrow
- Skin biopsy and fibroblast cultivation for specific enzyme testing
- Specific DNA testing.

Treatment

In the middle of the 20th century the principal treatment for some of the amino acid disorders was restriction of dietary protein and all other care was simply management of complications. In the last two decades, enzyme replacement, gene transfer, and organ transplantation have become available and beneficial for many previously untreatable disorders. Some of the more common or promising therapies are listed:

- Dietary restriction;
  - — E.g., reduction of dietary protein remains a mainstay of treatment for phenylketonuria and other amino acid disorders
- Dietary supplementation or replacement;
  - — E.g., oral ingestion of cornstarch several times a day helps prevent people with glycogen storage diseases from becoming seriously hypoglycemic.
- Vitamins;
  - — E.g., thiamine supplementation benefits several types of disorders that cause lactic acidosis.
- Intermediary metabolites, compounds, or drugs that facilitate or retard specific metabolic pathways
- Dialysis
- Enzyme replacement E.g. Acid-alpha glucosidase for Pompe disease
- Gene transfer
- Bone marrow or organ transplantation
- Treatment of symptoms and complications
- Prenatal diagnosis and avoidance of pregnancy or abortion of an affected fetus.

Chapter 3

Computational Neurogenetic Modelling

Computational neurogenetic modelling (CNGM) is concerned with the study and development of dynamic neuronal models for modelling brain functions with respect to genes and dynamic interactions between genes. These include neural network models and their integration with gene network models. This area brings together knowledge from various scientific disciplines, such as computer and information science, neuroscience and cognitive science, genetics and molecular biology, as well as engineering.

Mind Uploading

Mind uploading or whole brain emulation (sometimes called mind transfer) is the hypothetical process of scanning and mapping a biological brain in detail and copying its state into a computer system or another computational device. The computer would have to run a simulation model so faithful to the original that it would behave in essentially the same way as the original brain, or for all practical purposes, indistinguishably. The simulated mind is assumed to be part of a virtual reality simulated world, supported by an anatomic 3D body simulation model. Alternatively, the simulated mind could be assumed to reside in a computer inside (or connected to) a humanoid robot or a biological body, replacing its brain.

Whole brain emulation is discussed as a "logical endpoint" of the topical computational neuroscience and neuroinformatics fields, both about brain simulation for medical research purposes. It is discussed in artificial intelligence research publications as an approach to strong AI. Among futurists and within the transhumanist movement it is an important proposed life extension technology, originally suggested in biomedical literature in 1971. It is a central conceptual feature of numerous science fiction novels and films.

Whole brain emulation is considered by some scientists as a theoretical and futuristic but possible technology, although mainstream research funders and scientific journals remain skeptical. Several contradictory and already passed attempts have been made during the years to predict when whole human brain emulation can be achieved. Substantial mainstream research and development are however being done in relevant areas including development of faster super computers, virtual reality, brain-computer interfaces, animal brain mapping and simulation, and information extraction from dynamically functioning brains.

The question whether an emulated brain can be a human mind is debated by philosophers, and may be contradicted by the dualistic view of the human mind that is common in many religions.

Overview

The human brain contains about 100 billion nerve cells called neurons, each individually linked to other neurons by way of connectors called axons and dendrites. Signals at the junctures (synapses) of these connections are transmitted by the release and detection of chemicals known as neurotransmitters. The established neuroscientific consensus is that the human mind is largely an emergent property of the information processing of this neural network.

Importantly, neuroscientists have stated that important functions performed by the mind, such as learning, memory, and consciousness, are due to purely physical and electrochemical processes in the brain and are governed by applicable laws. For example, Christof Koch and Giulio Tononi wrote in IEEE Spectrum:

> *"Consciousness is part of the natural world. It depends, we believe, only on mathematics and logic and on the imperfectly known laws of physics, chemistry, and biology; it does not arise from some magical or otherworldly quality."*

The concept of mind uploading is based on this mechanistic view of the mind, and denies the vitalist view of human life and consciousness.

Many eminent computer scientists and neuroscientists have predicted that computers will be capable of thought and even attain consciousness, including Koch and Tononi, Douglas Hofstadter, Jeff Hawkins, Marvin Minsky, Randal A. Koene, and Rodolfo Llinas.

Such a machine intelligence capability might provide a computational substrate necessary for uploading.

However, even though uploading is dependent upon such a general capability it is conceptually distinct from general forms of AI in that it results from dynamic reanimation of information derived from a specific human mind so that the mind retains a sense of historical identity (other forms are possible but would compromise or eliminate the life-extension feature generally associated with uploading). The transferred and reanimated information would become a form of artificial intelligence, sometimes called an infomorph or "*noomorph.*"

Even if uploading is theoretically possible, the amount of storage and computational power required are difficult to predict. Nevertheless, many theorists have presented models of the brain and have established a range of estimates of the amount of computing power needed for partial and complete simulations (citations needed for Boahen, Modha, Izhikevich, Bostrom and Sandberg, others). Using these models, some have estimated that uploading may become possible within decades if trends such as Moore's Law continue.

The prospect of uploading human consciousness in this manner raises many philosophical questions involving identity, individuality and the soul, as well as numerous problems of medical ethics and morality of the process.

Theoretical Benefits

Immortality/Backup

In theory, if the information and processes of the mind can be disassociated from the biological body, they are no longer tied to the individual limits and lifespan of that body. Furthermore, information within a brain could be partly or wholly copied or transferred to one or more other substrates (including digital storage or another brain), thereby reducing or eliminating mortality risk. This general proposal appears to have been first made in the biomedical literature in 1971 by biogerontologist George M. Martin of the University of Washington.

Speedup

A computer-based intelligence such as an upload could potentially think much faster than a human even if it were no more intelligent. Human neurons exchange electrochemical signals with a maximum speed of about 150 meters per second, whereas the speed of light is about 300 million meters per second, about two million times faster. Also, neurons can generate a maximum of about 200 to 1000 action potentials or "spikes" per second, whereas the number of signals per second in modern computer chips is about 2 GHz (about ten million times greater) and expected to increase by at least a factor 100. Therefore, even if the computer components responsible for simulating a brain were not significantly smaller than a biological brain, and even if the temperature of these components was not significantly lower, Eliezer Yudkowsky of the Singularity Institute for Artificial Intelligence calculates a theoretical upper bound for the speed of a future artificial neural network. It could in theory run about 1 million times faster than a real brain, experiencing about a year of subjective time in only 31 seconds of real time.

However, in practice this massively parallel implementation would require separate computational units for each of the hundred billion neurons and each of the hundred trillion synapses. That requires an enormously large computer or artificial neural network in comparison with today's super-computers. In a less futuristic implementation, time-sharing would allow several neurons to be emulated sequentially by the same computational unit. Thus the size of the computer would be restricted, but the speedup would be lower. Assuming that cortical minicolumns organized into hypercolumns are the computational units, mammal brains can be emulated by today's super computers, but with slower speed than in a biological brain.

Multiple/Parallel Existence

Another concept explored in science fiction is the idea of more than one running "copy" of a human mind existing at once. Such copies could potentially allow an "individual" to experience many things at once, and later integrate the experiences of all copies into a central mentality at some point in the future, effectively allowing a single sentient being to "be many places at once" and "do many things at once"; this concept has been explored in fiction. Such partial and complete copies of a sentient being raise interesting questions regarding identity and individuality.

Relevant Technologies and Techniques

Computational Capacity

Advocates of mind uploading point to Moore's law to support the notion that the necessary computing power is expected to become available within a few decades. However, the actual computational requirements for running an uploaded human mind are very difficult to quantify, potentially rendering such an argument specious.

Regardless of the techniques used to capture or recreate the function of a human mind, the processing demands are likely to be immense, due to the large number of neurons in the human brain along with the considerable complexity of each neuron.

In 2004, Henry Markram, lead researcher of the "Blue Brain Project", has stated that "it is not [their] goal to build an intelligent neural network", based solely on the computational demands such a project would have.

It will be very difficult because, in the brain, every molecule is a powerful computer and we would need to simulate the structure and function of trillions upon trillions of molecules as well as all the rules that govern how they interact. You would literally need computers that are trillions of times bigger and faster than anything existing today.

Five years later, after successful simulation of part of a rat brain, the same scientist was much more bold and optimistic. In 2009, when he was director of the Blue Brain Project, he claimed that.

A detailed, functional artificial human brain can be built within the next 10 years.

Simulation Model Scale

Since the function of the human mind, and how it might arise from the working of the brain's neural network, are poorly understood issues, mind uploading relies on the idea of neural network emulation. Rather than having to understand the high-level psychological processes and large-scale structures of the brain, and model them using classical artificial intelligence methods and cognitive psychology models, the low-level structure of the underlying neural network is captured, mapped and emulated with a computer system. In computer science terminology, rather than analysing and reverse engineering the Behaviour of the algorithms and data structures that resides in the brain, a blueprint of its source code is translated to another programming language. The human mind and the personal identity then, theoretically, is generated by the emulated neural network in an identical fashion to it being generated by the biological neural network.

On the other hand, a molecule-scale simulation of the brain is not expected to be required, provided that the functioning of the neurons is not affected by quantum mechanical processes. The neural network emulation approach only requires that the functioning and interaction of neurons and synapses are understood. It is expected that it is sufficient with a black-box signal processing model of how the neurons respond to nerve impulses (electrical as well as chemical synaptic transmission).

A sufficiently complex and accurate model of the neurons is required. A traditional artificial neural network model, for example multi-layer perceptron network model, is not considered as sufficient. A dynamic spiking neural network model is required, which reflects that the neuron fires only when a membrane potential reaches a certain level. It is likely that the model must include delays, non-linear functions and differential equations describing the relation between electrophysical parameters such as electrical currents, voltages, membrane states (ion channel states) and neuromodulators.

Since learning and long-term memory are believed to result from strengthening or weakening the synapses via a mechanism known as synaptic plasticity or synaptic adaptation, the model should include this mechanism. The response of sensory receptors to various stimuli must also be modelled.

Furthermore, the model may have to include metabolism, i.e. how the neurons are affected by hormones and other chemical substances that may cross the blood-brain barrier. It is considered likely that the model must include currently unknown neuromodulators, neurotransmitters and ion channels. It is considered unlikely that the simulation model has to include protein interaction, which would make it computationally complex.

A digital computer simulation model of an analog system such as the brain is an approximation that introduces random quantization errors and distortion. However, the biological neurons also suffer from randomness and limited precision, for example due to background noise. The errors of the discrete model can be made smaller than the randomness of the biological brain by choosing a sufficiently high variable resolution and sample rate, and sufficiently accurate models of non-linearities. The computational power and computer memory must however be sufficient to run such large simulations, preferably in real time.

Scanning and Mapping Scale of an Individual

When modelling and simulating the brain of a specific individual, a brain map or connectivity database showing the connections between the neurons must be extracted from an anatomic model of the brain. This network map should show the connectivity of the whole nervous system, including the spinal cord, sensory receptors, and muscle cells.

Destructive scanning of the human brain including synaptic details is possible as of end of 2010. A full brain map should also reflect the synaptic strength (the "weight") of each connection. It is unclear if the current technology allows that.

It is proposed that short-term memory and working memory is prolonged or repeated firing of neurons, as well as intra-neural dynamic processes. Since the electrical and chemical signal state of the synapses and neurons may be hard to extract, the uploading might result in that the uploaded mind perceives a memory loss of the events immediately before the time of brain scanning.

A full brain map would occupy less than 2×10^{16} bytes (20000 Tb) and would store the addresses of the connected neurons, the synapse type and the synapse "weight" for each of the brains' 10^{15} synapses.

Serial Sectioning

A possible method for mind uploading is serial sectioning, in which the brain tissue and perhaps other parts of the nervous system are frozen and then scanned and analysed layer by layer, thus capturing the structure of the neurons and their interconnections. The exposed surface of frozen nerve tissue would be scanned and recorded, and then the surface layer of tissue removed. While this would be a very slow and labour intensive process, research is currently underway to automate the collection and microscopy of serial sections. The scans would then be analysed, and a model of the neural net recreated in the system that the mind was being uploaded into.

There are uncertainties with this approach using current microscopy techniques. If it is possible to replicate neuron function from its visible structure alone, then the resolution afforded by a scanning electron microscope would suffice for such a technique. However, as the function of brain tissue is partially determined by molecular events (particularly at synapses, but also at other places on the neuron's cell membrane), this may not suffice for capturing and simulating neuron functions. It may be possible to extend the techniques of serial sectioning and to capture the internal molecular makeup of neurons, through the use of sophisticated immunohistochemistry staining methods which could then be read via confocal laser scanning microscopy. However, as the physiological genesis of 'mind' is not currently known, this method may not be able to access all of the necessary biochemical information to recreate a human brain with sufficient fidelity.

Brain-computer Interfaces

Brain-computer interfaces (BCI) (also known as neuro-computer interfaces, direct neuron interfaces or cerebral interfaces) constitute one of the hypothetical technologies for the reading of information in the dynamically functioning brain. The production of this or a similar device may be essential to the possibility of mind uploading a living human subject.

Current Research

An artificial neural network almost half as complex as the brain of a mouse was run on an IBM blue gene supercomputer by a University of Nevada research team in 2007. A simulated time of one second took ten seconds of computer time. The researchers said they had seen "biologically consistent" nerve impulses flowed through the virtual cortex. However, the simulation lacked the structures seen in real mice brains, and they intend to improve the accuracy of the neuron model.

Blue Brain is a project, launched in May 2005 by IBM and the Swiss Federal Institute of Technology in Lausanne, with the aim to create a computer simulation of a mammalian cortical column, down to the molecular level. The project uses a supercomputer based on IBM's Blue Gene design to simulate the electrical Behaviour of neurons based upon their synaptic connectivity and complement of intrinsic membrane currents. The initial goal of the project, completed in December 2006, was the simulation of a rat neocortical column, which can be considered the smallest functional unit of the neocortex (the part of the brain thought to be responsible for higher functions such as conscious thought), containing 10,000 neurons (and 10^8 synapses). Between 1995 and 2005, Henry Markram mapped the types of neurons and their connections in such a column. In November 2007, the project reported the end of the first phase, delivering a data-driven process for creating, validating, and researching the neocortical column. The project seeks to eventually reveal aspects of human cognition and various psychiatric disorders caused by malfunctioning neurons, such as autism, and to understand how pharmacological agents affect network Behaviour. An organization called the Brain Preservation Foundation was founded in 2010 and is offering a Brain Preservation Technology prize to promote exploration of brain preservation technology in service of humanity. The Prize, presently $106,000, will be awarded in two parts, 25% to the first international team to preserve a whole mouse brain, and 75% to the first team to preserve a whole large animal brain in a manner that could also be adopted for humans in a hospital or hospice setting immediately upon clinical death. Ultimately the goal of this prize is to generate a whole brain map which may be used in support of separate efforts to upload and possibly 'reboot' a mind in virtual space.

Issues

Legal, Political and Economical Issues: It may be difficult for the society to supervise that human rights are not threatened in any computer in the world. It might for example be tempting for social science researchers to expose simulated minds, or whole isolated societies of simulated minds, to controlled experiments, where many copies of the same minds, or repeated reruns of the same simulation, are exposed to different test conditions.

The only limited physical resource to be expected in a simulated world is the computational capacity, meaning simulation speed. As speed depends on the availability of computing resources, wealthy, powerful or privileged individuals in a society of uploads might experience more subjective time than others in the same real time, or may be able to run copies of them selves or others, and thus produce more service and become even more wealthy. Others may suffer from computational resource starvation and show a slow motion Behaviour, unless prohibited by law.

Copying vs. Moving

Another philosophical issue with mind uploading is whether an uploaded mind is really the "same" sentience, or simply an exact copy with the same memories and personality; or, indeed, what the difference could be between such a copy and the original. This issue is especially complex if the original remains essentially unchanged by the procedure, thereby resulting in an obvious copy which could potentially have rights separate from the unaltered, obvious original.

Most projected brain scanning technologies, such as serial sectioning of the brain, would necessarily be destructive, and the original brain would not survive the brain scanning procedure. But if it can be kept intact, the computer-based consciousness could be a copy of the still-living biological person. It is in that case implicit that copying a consciousness could be as feasible as literally moving it into one or several copies, since these technologies generally involve simulation of a human brain in a computer of some sort, and digital files such as computer programs can be copied precisely. It is usually assumed that once the versions are exposed to different sensory inputs, their experiences would begin to diverge, but all their memories up until the moment of the copying would remain the same.

The problem is made even more serious by the possibility of creating a potentially infinite number of initially identical copies of the original person, which would of course all exist simultaneously as distinct beings. The most parsimonious view of this phenomenon is that the two (or more) minds would share memories of their past but from the point of duplication would simply be distinct minds (although this is complicated by merging). Many complex variations are possible.

Depending on computational capacity, the simulation may run at slower or faster simulation time as compared to the elapsed physical time, resulting in that the simulated mind would perceive that the physical world is running in slow motion or fast motion respectively, while biological persons will see the simulated mind in fast or slow motion respectively. A brain simulation can be started, paused, backed-up and rerun from a saved backup state at any time. The simulated mind would in the latter case forget everything that has happened after the instant of backup, and perhaps not even be aware that it is repeating itself. An older version of a simulated mind may meet a younger version and share experiences with it.

Bekenstein Bound

The Bekenstein bound is an upper limit on information that can be contained within a given finite region of space which has a finite amount of energy or, conversely, the maximum amount of information required to perfectly describe a given physical system down to the quantum level. An average human brain has a weight of 1.5 kg and a volume of 1260 cm^3. The energy ($E = m \cdot c^2$) will be $1.34813 \cdot 10^{17}$ J and if the brain is approximate to a sphere then the radius ($V = 4 \pi r^3/3$) will be $6.70030 \cdot 10^{-2}$ m. The Bekenstein bound ($I \leq 2 \pi r \cdot E' \cdot c \cdot \ln 2$) will be $2.58991 \cdot 10^{42}$ bit and represent an upper bound on the information needed to perfectly recreate the average human brain down to the quantum level. This implies that the number of different states ($\Omega = 2^I$) of the human brain (and of the mind if the physicalism is true) is at most $10^{7.79640 \cdot 1041}$.

However, as described above, many mind uploading advocates expect that quantum-level models and molecule-scale simulation of the neurons will not be needed, so the Bekenstein bound only represents a maximum upper limit.

Mind Uploading in Science Fiction

Mind Uploading Advocates and Critics

Followers of the Raëlian religion advocate mind uploading in the process of human cloning to achieve eternal life. Living inside of a computer is also seen by followers as an eminent possibility.

However, mind uploading is also advocated by a number of secular researchers in neuroscience and artificial intelligence, such as Marvin Minsky. In 1993, Joe Strout created a small web site called the Mind Uploading Home Page, and began advocating the idea in cryonics circles and elsewhere on the net. That site has not been actively updated in recent years, but it has spawned other sites including MindUploading.org, run by Randal A. Koene, Ph.D., who also moderates a mailing list on the topic. These advocates see mind uploading as a medical procedure which could eventually save countless lives.

Many transhumanists look forward to the development and deployment of mind uploading technology, with many predicting that it will become possible within the 21st century due to technological trends such as Moore's Law. Many view it as the end phase of the Transhumanist project, which might be said to begin with the genetic engineering of biological humans, continue with the cybernetic enhancement of genetically engineered humans, and finally obtain with the replacement of all remaining biological aspects.

The book *Beyond Humanity: CyberEvolution and Future Minds* by Gregory S. Paul & Earl D. Cox, is about the eventual (and, to the authors, almost inevitable) evolution of computers into sentient beings, but also deals with human mind transfer. Richard Doyle's *Wetwares: Experiments in PostVital Living* deals extensively with uploading from the perspective of distributed embodiment, arguing for example that humans are currently part of the "artificial life phenotype." Doyle's vision reverses the polarity on uploading, with artificial life forms such as uploads actively seeking out biological embodiment as part of their reproductive strategy. Raymond Kurzweil, a prominent advocate of transhumanism and the likelihood of a technological singularity, has suggested that the easiest path to human-level artificial intelligence may lie in "reverse-engineering the human brain", which he usually uses to refer to the creation of a new intelligence based on the general "principles of operation" of the brain, but he also sometimes uses the term to refer to the notion of uploading individual human minds based on highly detailed scans and simulations.

Brain-reading

Brain reading uses the responses of multiple voxels in the brain evoked by some stimulus and detected by fMRI in order to decode the stimulus. Brain reading studies differ in the type of decoding (classification, identification and reconstruction), the target of decoding (visual patterns, auditory patterns, cognitive states, etc.), and the decoding algorithms (linear classification, nonlinear classification, direct reconstruction, bayesian reconstruction, etc.).

Classification

In classification a pattern of activity across multiple voxels is used to determine the particular class from which the stimulus was drawn. Many studies have classified visual stimuli, but this approach has also been used to classify cognitive states.

Reconstruction

In reconstruction brain reading the aim is to create a literal picture of the image that was presented. Early studies used voxels from early visual cortex areas (V1, V2, and V3) to reconstruct geometric stimuli made up of flickering checkerboard patterns.

Natural Images

More recent studies used voxels from early and anterior visual cortex areas forward of them (visual areas V3A, V3B, V4, and the lateral occipital) together with Bayesian inference techniques to reconstruct complex natural images. This brain reading approach uses three components: A structural encoding model that characterizes responses in early visual areas; a semantic encoding model that characterizes responses in anterior visual areas; and a Bayseian prior that describes the distribution of structural and semantic scene statistics. Experimentally the procedure is for subjects to view 1750 black and white natural images that are correlated with voxel activation in their brains. Then subjects viewed another 120 novel target images, and information from the earlier scans is used reconstruct them. Natural images used include pictures of a seaside cafe and harbour, performers on a stage, and dense foliage.

Other Types

It is possible to track which of two forms of rivalrous binocular illusions a person was subjectively experiencing from fMRI signals. The category of event which a person freely recalls can be identified from fMRI before they say what they remembered. Statistical analysis of EEG brainwaves has been claimed to allow the recognition of phonemes, and at a 60% to 75% level colour and visual shape words.

Accuracy

Brain-reading accuracy is increasing steadily as the quality of the data and the complexity of the decoding algorithms improve. In one recent experiment it was possible to identify which single image was being seen from a set of 120. In another it was possible to correctly identify 90% of the time which of two categories the stimulus came and the specific semantic category (out of 23) of the target image 40% of the time.

Limitations

It has been noted that so far that brain reading is limited. "in practice exact reconstructions are impossible to achieve by any reconstruction algorithm on the basis of brain activity signals acquired by fMRI. This is because all reconstructions will inevitably be limited by inaccuracies in the encoding models and noise in the measured signals. Our results demonstrate that the natural image prior is a powerful (if unconventional) tool for mitigating the effects of these fundamental limitations. A natural image prior with only six million images is sufficient to produce reconstructions that are structurally and semantically similar to a target image."

Brain Fingerprinting

"Brain Fingerprinting" is exactly identical to standard P300 lie detection using David Lykken's "Guilty Knowledge Test", except that it also uses other brainwaves in addition to P300. Only one study— has ever tested its accuracy, and that laboratory study by "Brain Fingerprinting"'s developer used only 6 participants (3 "guilty" and 3 "innocent"), rendering any conclusions drawn therefrom statistically insignificant (psychologists typically require 3 sigma and n=15 for minimal statistical significance). The citations in the rest of this article, particularly to the work of Iacono, are mis-attributed and refer to studies of the P300 GKT method alone, not to Farwell's "Brain Fingerprinting." P300 measurement of the GKT "orienting reflex" is as accurate as polygraph measurement of the orienting reflex, and there is no logical reason to believe (and no (good) scientific studies to demonstrate) that using other brainwaves in addition to P300 will improve the test, as the problem isn't measuring the physiological "orienting reflex" response but in formulating the right questions and alternatives for the situation.

Brain Fingerprinting is a controversial forensic science technique that uses brain-reading techniques to determine whether specific information is stored in a subject's brain. It does this by measuring electrical brainwave responses to words, phrases, or pictures that are presented on a computer screen. Brain fingerprinting was invented by Lawrence Farwell. The theory is that the brain processes known, relevant information differently from the way it processes unknown or irrelevant information. The brain's processing of known information, such as the details of a crime stored in the brain, is revealed by a specific pattern in the EEG (electroencephalograph). Farwell's brain fingerprinting originally used the well known P300 brain response to detect the brain's recognition of the known information.

Later Farwell discovered the MERMER ("Memory and Encoding Related Multifaceted Electroencephalographic Response"), which includes the P300 and additional features and is reported to provide a higher level of accuracy than the P300 alone. In peer-reviewed publications Farwell and colleagues report over 99% accuracy in laboratory research and real-life field applications. In independent research William Iacono and others who followed identical or similar scientific protocols to Farwell's have reported a similar high level of accuracy.

Brain fingerprinting has been applied in a number of high-profile criminal cases, including helping to catch serial killer JB Grinder (Dalbey 1999) and to exonerate innocent convict Terry Harrington after he had been falsely convicted of murder (Harrington v. State). Brain fingerprinting has been ruled admissible in court. In the controversial Sister Abhaya murder case, the Ernakulam Chief Judicial Magistrate court had asked the Central Bureau of Investigation to make use of all modern investigation techniques, including brain fingerprinting.

Brain fingerprinting technique has been criticized on a number of fronts. Although independent scientists who have used the same or similar methods as Farwell's brain fingerprinting have achieved similar, highly accurate results, different methods have yielded different results. J. Peter Rosenfeld used P300-based tests incorporating fundamentally different methods, resulting in as low as chance accuracy as well as susceptibility to countermeasures, and criticized brain fingerprinting based on the premise that the shortcomings of his alternative technique should generalize to all other techniques in which the P300 is among the brain responses measured, including brain fingerprinting.

Brain Fingerprinting was an international finalist in the Global Security Challenge 2008 in London.

Technique

The technique uses the well known fact that an electrical signal known as P300 is emitted from an individual's brain beginning approximately 300 milliseconds after it is confronted with a stimulus of special significance, e.g. a rare vs. a common stimulus or a stimulus the subject is asked to count. The application of this in brain fingerprinting is to detect the P300 as a response to stimuli related to the crime or other investigated situation, e.g., a murder weapon, victim's face, or knowledge of the internal workings of a terrorist cell. Because it is based on EEG signals, the system does not require the subject to issue verbal responses to questions or stimuli.

The person to be tested wears a special headband with electronic sensors that measure the EEG from several locations on the scalp. The subject views stimuli consisting of words, phrases, or pictures presented on a computer screen. Stimuli are of three types: 1) "irrelevant" stimuli that are irrelevant to the investigated situation and to the test subject, 2) "target" stimuli that are relevant to the investigated situation and are known to the subject, and 3) "probe" stimuli that are relevant to the investigated situation and that the subject denies knowing. Probes contain information that is known only to the perpetrator and investigators, and not to the general public or to an innocent suspect who was not at the scene of the crime. Before the test, the scientist identifies the targets to the subject, and makes sure that he/she knows these relevant stimuli. The scientist also makes sure that the subject does not know the probes for any reason unrelated to the crime, and that the subject denies knowing the probes. The subject is told why the probes are significant, but is not told which items are the probes and which are irrelevant.

Since brain fingerprinting uses cognitive brain responses, brain fingerprinting does not depend on the emotions of the subject, nor is it affected by emotional responses. Brain fingerprinting is fundamentally different from the polygraph (lie-detector), which measures emotion-based physiological signals such as heart rate, sweating, and blood pressure (Farwell 1994). Also, unlike polygraph testing, it does not attempt to determine whether or not the subject is lying or telling the truth. Rather, it measures the subject's brain response to relevant words, phrases, or pictures to detect whether or not the relevant information is stored in the subject's brain.

By comparing the responses to the different types of stimuli, the brain fingerprinting system mathematically computes a determination of "information present" (the subject knows the crime-relevant information contained in the probe stimuli) or "information absent" (the subject does not know the information) and a statistical confidence for the determination. This determination is mathematically computed, and does not involve the subjective judgment of the scientist.

Background and Terminology

"Brain fingerprinting" is a computer-based test that is designed to discover, document, and provide evidence of guilty knowledge regarding crimes, and to identify individuals with a specific training or expertise such as members of dormant terrorist cells or bomb makers. It has also been used to evaluate brain functioning as a means of early detection of Alzheimer's and other cognitively degenerative diseases, and to evaluate the effectiveness of advertising by measuring brain responses.

The technique is described in Dr. Farwell's paper "Using Brain MERMER Testing to Detect Concealed Knowledge Despite Efforts to Conceal", published in the Journal of Forensic Sciences in 2001 by Dr. Farwell and FBI Supervisory Special Agent Sharon Smith of the FBI.

The paper describes a test of brain fingerprinting, a technology based on EEG that is purported to be able to detect the existence of prior knowledge or memory in the brain. The P300 occurs when the tested subject is presented with a rarely occurring stimulus that is significant in context (for example, in the context of a crime). When an irrelevant stimulus is presented, a P300 is not expected to occur. The P300 is widely known in the scientific community, and is also known as an oddball-evoked P300.

While researching the P300, Dr. Farwell created a more detailed test that not only includes the P300, but also observes the stimulus response up to 1400 ms after the stimulus. He calls this brain response a MERMER, memory and encoding related multifaceted electroencephalographic response. The P300, an electrically positive component, is maximal at the midline parietal area of the head and has a peak latency of approximately 300 to 800 ms. The MERMER includes the P300 and also includes an electrically negative component, with an onset latency of approximately 800-1200ms. According to Dr. Farwell, the MERMER includes additional features involving changes in the frequency of the EEG signal, but for the purposes of signal detection and practical application the MERMER is sufficiently characterized by the P300 and the following negative component in the brain response.

Current uses and Research

Brain Fingerprinting has two primary applications: 1) detecting the record of a specific crime, terrorist act, or incident stored in the brain, and 2) detecting a specific type of knowledge, expertise, or training, such as knowledge specific to FBI agents, Al-Qaeda-trained terrorists, or bomb makers.

The seminal paper by Dr. Farwell and Emmanuel Donchin reported successful application of the technique in detecting knowledge of both laboratory mock crimes and real-life events, with no false positives and no false negatives.

In a study with the FBI, Dr. Farwell and FBI scientist Drew Richardson, former chief of the FBI's chem-bio-nuclear counterterrorism unit, used brain fingerprinting to show that test subjects from specific groups could be identified by detecting specific knowledge which would only be known to members of those groups. A group of 17 FBI agents and 4 non-agents were exposed to stimuli (words, phrases, and acronyms) that were flashed on a computer screen. The probe stimuli contained information that would be common knowledge only to someone with FBI training. Brain fingerprinting correctly distinguished the FBI agents from the non-agents.

The CIA has also funded Farwell's research (Dale 2001). In a study funded by the CIA, Farwell and colleagues used brain fingerprinting to detect which individuals had US Navy military medical training. All 30 subjects were correctly determined to have or not to have the specific information regarding military medicine stored in their brains. In another CIA-funded study, brain fingerprinting correctly detected which individuals had participated in specific real-life events, some of which were crimes, based on the record stored in their brains. Accuracy again was 100%. Dr. Farwell collaborated with FBI scientist Sharon Smith in a further study in which brain fingerprinting detected real-life events that was published in the *Journal of Forensic Sciences*.

In another CIA-funded study, a group of subjects enacted a simulated espionage scenario and were then tested on relevant stimuli in the form of pictorial probes. Brain fingerprinting correctly identified all individuals who were "information present" and "information absent".

Use in Criminal Investigation

Farwell's brain fingerprinting has been ruled admissible as evidence in court in the reversal of the murder conviction of Terry Harrington. Following a hearing on post-conviction relief on November 14, 2000, an Iowa District Court held that Dr. Farwell's brain fingerprinting P-300 test results were admissible as scientific evidence as defined in Congress Ruling 702 and in the Daubert standard. Harrington was freed by the Iowa Supreme Court on grounds.

Based on two days of testimony from expert witnesses on both sides of the issue and hundreds of pages of supporting documentation, brain fingerprinting was ruled admissible in the Harrington case (Harrington v. State). In order to be ruled admissible under the prevailing Daubert standard established by the US Supreme Court, the Court required proof that brain fingerprinting is 1) tested and proven, 2) peer reviewed and published, 3) accurate and systematically applied, and 4) well accepted in the relevant scientific community. In ruling brain fingerprinting admissible as scientific evidence, the Court stated the following:

> *"In the spring of 2000, Harrington was given a test by Dr. Lawrence Farwell. The test is based on a 'P300 effect'."*
>
> *"The P-300 effect has been recognized for nearly twenty years."*
>
> *"The P-300 effect has been subject to testing and peer review in the scientific community."*
>
> *"The consensus in the community of psycho-physiologists is that the P300 effect is valid."*
>
> *"The evidence resulting from Harrington's 'brain fingerprinting' test was discovered after the fact. It is newly discovered."*

Limitations of brain Fingerprinting

Both the strengths and limitations of brain fingerprinting are documented in detail in the expert witness testimony of Dr. Farwell and two other expert witnesses in the Harrington case (Harrington v. State) and in a Law Enforcement Technology article (Simon 2005) as well as in Farwell's publications and patents. The limitations of brain fingerprinting described below are also summarized in PBS 2004, PBS Innovation Series – "Brain Fingerprinting: Ask the Experts".

Brain fingerprinting detects information-processing brain responses that reveal what information is stored in the subject's brain. It does not detect how that information got there. This fact has implications for how and when the technique can be applied. In a case where a suspect claims not to have been at the crime scene and has no legitimate reason for knowing the details of the crime, and investigators have information that has not been released to the public, brain fingerprinting can determine objectively whether or not the subject possesses that information. In such a case, brain fingerprinting could provide useful evidence.

If, however, the suspect knows everything that the investigators know about the crime for some legitimate reason, then the test cannot be applied. There are several circumstances in which this may be the case. If a suspect acknowledges being at the scene of the crime, but claims to be a witness and not a perpetrator, then the fact that he knows details about the crime would not be incriminating. There would be no reason to conduct a test, because the resulting "information present" response would simply show that the suspect knew the details about the crime – knowledge which he already admits and which he gained at the crime scene whether he was a witness or a perpetrator. Another case where brain fingerprinting is not applicable would be one wherein a suspect and an alleged victim – say, of an alleged sexual assault – agree on the details of what was said and done, but disagree on the intent of the parties. Brain fingerprinting detects only information, and not intent. The fact that the suspect knows the uncontested facts of the circumstance does not tell us which party's version of the intent is correct.

In a case where the suspect knows everything that the investigators know because he has been exposed to all available information in a previous trial, there is no available information with which to construct probe stimuli, so a test cannot be conducted. Even in a case where the suspect knows many of the details about the crime, however, it is sometimes possible to discover salient information that the perpetrator must have encountered in the course of committing the crime, but the suspect claims not to know and would not know if he were innocent. This was the case with Terry Harrington (Harrington v. State). By examining reports, interviewing witnesses, and visiting the crime scene and surrounding areas, Dr. Farwell was able to discover salient features of the crime that Harrington had never been exposed to at his previous trials. The brain fingerprinting test showed that the record in Harrington's brain did not contain these salient features of the crime, but only the details about the crime that he had learned after the fact.

Obviously, in structuring a brain fingerprinting test, a scientist must avoid including information that has been made public. Detecting that a suspect knows information he obtained by reading a newspaper would not be of use in a criminal investigation, and standard brain fingerprinting procedures eliminate all such information from the structuring of a test. News accounts containing many of the details of a crime do not interfere with the development of a brain fingerprinting test, however; they simply limit the material that can be tested. Even in highly publicized cases, there are almost always many details that are known to the investigators but not released to the public (Simon 2005), and these can be used as stimuli to test the subject for knowledge that he would have no way to know except by committing the crime.

Another situation where brain fingerprinting is not applicable is one where the authorities have no information about what crime may have taken place. For example, an individual may disappear under circumstances where a specific suspect had a strong motive to murder the individual. Without any evidence, authorities do not know whether a murder took place, or the individual decided to take a trip and tell no one, or some other criminal or non-criminal event happened. If there is no known information on which a suspect could be tested, a brain fingerprinting test cannot be structured.

Similarly, brain fingerprinting is not applicable for general screening, for example, in general pre-employment or employee screening wherein any number of undesirable activities or intentions may be relevant. If the investigators have no idea what crime or undesirable act the individual may have committed, there is no way to structure appropriate stimuli to detect the telltale knowledge that would result from committing the crime. Brain fingerprinting can, however, be used for specific screening or focused screening, when investigators have some idea what they are looking for. For example, brain fingerprinting can be used to detect whether a person has knowledge that would identify him as an FBI agent, an Al-Qaeda-trained terrorist, a member of a criminal organization or terrorist cell, or a bomb maker (Farwell *et al.* 2006).

Brain fingerprinting does not detect lies. It simply detects information. No questions are asked or answered during a brain fingerprinting test. The subject neither lies nor tells the truth during a brain fingerprinting test, and the outcome of the test is unaffected by whether he has lied or told the truth at any other time. The outcome of "information present" or "information absent" depends on whether the relevant information is stored in the brain, and not on what the subject says about it.

Brain fingerprinting does not determine whether a suspect is guilty or innocent of a crime. This is a legal determination to be made by a judge and jury, not a scientific determination to be made by a computer or a scientist. Brain fingerprinting can provide scientific evidence that the judge and jury can weigh along with the other evidence in reaching their decisions regarding the crime. To remain within the realm of scientific testimony, however, a brain fingerprinting expert witness must testify only regarding the scientific test and information stored in the brain revealed by the test, as Dr. Farwell did in the Harrington case (Harrington v. State). Like the testimony of other forensic scientists, a brain fingerprinting scientist's testimony does not include interpreting the scientific evidence in terms of guilt or innocence. A DNA expert may testify that two DNA samples match, one from the crime scene and one from the suspect, but he does not conclude "this man is a murderer." Similarly, a brain fingerprinting expert can testify to the outcome of the test that the subject has specific information stored in his brain about the crime (or not), but the interpretation of this evidence in terms of guilt or innocence is solely up to the judge and jury.

Just as all witness testimony depends on the memory of the witness, brain fingerprinting depends on the memory of the subject. Like all witness testimony, brain fingerprinting results must be viewed in light of the limitations on human memory and the factors affecting it. Brain fingerprinting can provide scientific evidence regarding what information is stored in a subject's brain. It does not determine what information *should be*, *could be*, or *would be* stored in the subject's brain if the subject were innocent or guilty. It only measures what actually *is* stored in the brain. How this evidence is interpreted, and what conclusions are drawn based on it, is outside the realm of the science and the scientist. This is up to the judge and jury. It is up to the prosecutor and the defence attorney to argue, and the judge and jury to decide, the significance and weight of the brain fingerprinting evidence in making a determination of whether or not the subject committed the crime.

Like all forensic science techniques, brain fingerprinting depends on the evidence-gathering process which lies outside the realm of science to provide the evidence to be scientifically tested. Before a brain fingerprinting test can be conducted, an investigator must discover relevant information about the crime or investigated situation. This investigative process, in which the investigator gathers the information to be tested from the crime scene or other sources related to the crime, depends on the skill and judgment of the investigator. This process is outside the scientific process; it precedes the scientific process of brain fingerprinting. This investigative process produces the probe stimuli to be tested. Brain fingerprinting science only determines whether the information tested is stored in the brain of the subject or not. It does not provide scientific data on the effectiveness of the investigation that produced the information about the crime that was tested. In this regard, brain fingerprinting is similar to other forensic sciences. A DNA test determines only whether two DNA samples match, it does not determine whether the investigator did an effective job of collecting DNA from the crime scene. Similarly, a brain fingerprinting test determines only whether or not the information stored in the suspect's brain matches the information contained in the probe stimuli. This is information that the investigator provided to the scientist to test scientifically, based on the investigative process that is outside the realm of science. In making their determination about the crime and the suspect's possible role in it, the judge and jury must take into account not only the scientific determination of "information present" or "information absent" provided by the brain fingerprinting test; they must also make common-sense, human, non-scientific judgments regarding the information gathered by the investigator and to what degree knowledge or lack of knowledge of that information sheds light on the suspect's possible role in the crime. Brain fingerprinting is not a substitute for effective investigation on the part of the investigator or for common sense and good judgment on the part of the judge and jury (PBS 2004).

Future Applications and Research

After Dr. Farwell invented Brain Fingerprinting, he withheld it from the public for 15 years while he, his colleagues, and other, independent scientists tested it in the laboratory and in the field. Farwell's decision to apply this science in real-life situations has been controversial (Dale 2001). In the years since Dr. Farwell first began applying the technology in the real world, proponents, including other scientists who have successfully applied the technique such as FBI scientist Drew Richardson, and those who have been freed or otherwise helped by brain fingerprinting, have advocated continuing and expanded application of the technology in the real world. Critics, including some scientists, and those whose criminal activities have been thwarted by brain fingerprinting have advocated further delay in applying the technique.

According to sworn testimony by Dr. William Iacono, an independent expert unaffiliated with Dr. Farwell who has conducted extensive research in the area, the science underlying brain fingerprinting has been published in hundreds, perhaps thousands, of articles in the scientific literature, and the specific application of this science in detecting information has been published in about 50 studies (Harrington v. State). Although the science is well established, opinions among scientists and others on the social policy question of how and when this science should be applied vary widely. Dr. Farwell's decision to apply this science in bringing criminals to justice (Dalbey 1999) and freeing innocent suspects (Harrington v. State) is controversial. Various other attempts to apply this science in the detection of concealed information have varied in accuracy and efficacy, depending on the scientific procedures used (Harrington v. State).

Farwell and colleagues as well as other, independent scientists who have precisely replicated Farwell's research or used similar methods, have obtained accuracy rates approaching 100% in both laboratory and field conditions.

Different scientific methods, however, have yielded different results. In P300-based tests using different experimental methods, different brain responses, different stimulus types, different data collection methods, different analysis methods, and different statistics from those used in Farwell's brain fingerprinting, Rosenfeld reported accuracy rates close to those obtained by chance, even without countermeasures. Moreover, Rosenfeld's alternative technique proved susceptible to countermeasures.

Controversy has arisen over the best explanation for the fact that Farwell and others who use similar scientific methods have achieved near-100% accuracy, while Rosenfeld's alternative method yielded variable accuracy, sometimes as low as chance.

Farwell, FBI scientists Drew Richardson and Sharon Smith, and other brain fingerprinting experts claim that one cannot necessarily expect to obtain the same accuracy as brain fingerprinting without following standard brain fingerprinting scientific protocols or similar methods, that Rosenfeld's failure to achieve accuracy rates comparable to those of brain fingerprinting is the result of the substantial differences in scientific methodology between his alternative technique and brain fingerprinting, and therefore the fact that Rosenfeld's alternative technique is admittedly inaccurate and susceptible to countermeasures is no reflection on brain fingerprinting.

Proponents advocate continuing the use of brain fingerprinting to bring criminals and terrorists to justice and to free innocent suspects, while at the same time more research is continuing. Dr. Farwell and former FBI scientist Dr. Drew Richardson are among the scientists who advocate continuing the use of brain fingerprinting in criminal investigations and counterterrorism, without delay, as well as ongoing research on the technology.

Dr. Farwell was interviewed by *TIME* magazine after he was selected to the TIME 100: The Next Wave, the 100 innovators who may be "the Picassos or Einsteins of the 21st Century." He said, "The fundamental task in law enforcement and espionage and counterespionage is to determine the truth. My philosophy is that there is a tremendous cost in failing to apply the technology." (Dale 2001)

Critics of brain fingerprinting claim that the inaccuracy and susceptibility to countermeasures of Rosenfeld's alternative technique also cast doubt on all P300-based information-detection techniques, including brain fingerprinting (Rosenfeld 2005). Critics agree with proponents that ongoing research on brain fingerprinting is valuable and desirable. Unlike proponents, however, critics advocate a discontinuation of the use of brain fingerprinting in criminal and counterterrorism cases while this research is continuing.

A report by the United States General Accounting Office (now called Government Accountability Office) in 2001 reported that the scientists it interviewed (including Farwell, Iacono, Richardson, Rosenfeld, Smith, Donchin, and others) all had expressed a need for more research to investigate brain fingerprinting's application as forensic science tool (Initial GAO Report). While they were unanimous in their support of more scientific research, scientists and others expressed widely varying views on the social policy question of whether brain fingerprinting should continue to be applied to bring criminals and terrorists to justice and to free innocent suspects while this research continues. The initial GAO report was completed before the terrorist attacks of 9/11/2001, when the primary interest of federal agencies in detection methods was for employee screening, rather than detecting terrorists. (As discussed above, brain fingerprinting is not applicable in general employee screening.) Senator Charles Grassley, who commissioned the initial report, has asked the GAO produce a new report that examines the value of brain fingerprinting in counterterrorism and criminal investigations in the post-911 world in light of published scientific research on the application of the technique in the laboratory and the field (Fox 2006a).

Brain Mapping

Brain mapping is a set of neuroscience techniques predicated on the mapping of (biological) quantities or properties onto spatial representations of the (human or non-human) brain resulting in maps.

Overview

All neuroimaging can be considered part of brain mapping. Brain mapping can be conceived as a higher form of neuroimaging, producing brain images supplemented by the result of additional (imaging or non-imaging) data processing or analysis, such as maps projecting (measures of) behaviour onto brain regions. Brain Mapping techniques are constantly evolving, and rely on the development and refinement of image acquisition, representation, analysis, visualization and interpretation techniques. Functional and structural neuroimaging are at the core of the mapping aspect of Brain Mapping.

History

In the late 1980s in the United States, the Institute of Medicine of the National Academy of Science was commissioned to establish a panel to investigate the value of integrating neuroscientific information across a variety of techniques.

Of specific interest is using structural and functional magnetic resonance imaging (fMRI), electroencephalography (EEG), positron emission tomography (PET) and other non-invasive scanning techniques to map anatomy, physiology, perfusion, function and phenotypes of the human brain. Both healthy and diseased brains may be mapped to study memory, learning, aging, and drug effects in various populations such as people with schizophrenia, autism, and clinical depression. This led to the establishment of the Human Brain Project. Following a series of meetings, the International Consortium for Brain Mapping (ICBM) evolved. The ultimate goal is to develop flexible computational brain atlases.

On 5.5.2010 the Supreme Court in India in its historical judgement on several PIL's has declared brain mapping,lie detector test and narcoanalysis as unconstitutional as it violates Article 20 (3)of Fundamental Rights.It cannot be conducted forcefully on any individual and requires one's consent for the same when it is conducted with one's consent the material so obtained will be regarded as evidence during trial of cases according to Section 27 of Evidence Act.

Current Atlas Tools

- Talairach Atlas, 1988
- Harvard Whole Brain Atlas, 1995
- MNI Template, 1998 (The standard template of SPM and International Consortium for Brain Mapping).

Bioinformatics Companies

This is a list of bioinformatics companies.

- Accelrys
- AstraZeneca
- BIOBASE provides biological databases, bioinformatics solutions for expression data, promoter and pathway analysis and KPO services
- Biomatters Ltd. is the New Zealand-based company that creates the Geneious software suite.
- Biomax Informatics AG bioinformatics services and solutions
- CLC Bio free Bioinformatics workbenches.
- DNASTAR provides DNA sequence assembly and analysis, including Sanger and next generation sequence assembly and gene expression analysis.
- Gene Codes Corporation
- Genedata provides software products and services for data analysis and storage in Transcriptomics, Toxicogenomics, High-throughput screening (HTS), Genomics and related disciplines.
- Geneious combines many DNA and protein sequence analysis tools.
- Genomatix offering biology driven analysis pipelines for microarray analysis, ChIP on Chip and Solexa/454 data. Multiple tools and databases for analysis of gene regulation. Comparative genomics and most complete and quality checked genomic annotation for 17 species.
- Genostar provides streamlined bioinformatics solutions: sequence assembly, mapping, annotation transfer and identification of protein domains, comparative genomics, structural searches, metabolic pathway analysis, modelling and simulation of biological networks

- Ingenuity Systems is a provider of information solutions and custom services for life science researchers, computational biologists and bioinformaticists, and life science industry suppliers
- Inte:Ligand
- Korea Computer Centre Sinhung Company
- MacVector, providing MacVector and Assembler. MacVector is a Macintosh application that provides sequence editing, primer design, internet database searching, protein analysis, sequence confirmation, multiple sequence alignment, phylogenetic reconstruction, coding region analysis, and a wide variety of other functions.
- PREMIER Biosoft International is a bioinformatics company with an expertise in software development, marketing and bioinformatics consultancy for in-silico experiment design. PREMIER Biosoft has authored software for pcr primer & probe design, microarray design, glycan structure identificatin, plasmid map drawing and tissue microarray data analysis.
- Qlucore Qlucore Omics Explorer is a bioinformatics software program.
- Rosetta Biosoftware
- SimBioSys develops the eHITS software for molecular docking (flexible ligand docking & fast pre-docking), pharmacophore modelling, de novo design and retrosynthetic analysis software tools
- Strand Life Sciences offers solutions for micro array gene expression analysis, computational chemistry, data analysis and visualizations.
- VADLO Search engine for bioinformatics software, databases and online tools.

Health Informatics

Health informatics (also called health care informatics, healthcare informatics, medical informatics or biomedical informatics) is a discipline at the intersection of information science, computer science, and health care. It deals with the resources, devices, and methods required to optimize the acquisition, storage, retrieval, and use of information in health and biomedicine.

Health informatics tools include not only computers but also clinical guidelines, formal medical terminologies, and information and communication systems. It is applied to the areas of nursing, clinical care, dentistry, pharmacy, public health, occupational therapy, and (bio)medical research. Two primary considerations in health informatics are the creation of data with accuracy sufficient to support reliable public health science; and at the same time protect the privacy and civil liberties of the recipients of health care services.

Aspects of the field :

- architectures for electronic medical records and other health information systems used for billing, scheduling, and research
- decision support systems in healthcare, including clinical decision support systems and information workflows
- standards (e.g. DICOM, HL7) and integration profiles (e.g. Integrating the Healthcare Enterprise) to facilitate the exchange of information between healthcare information systems- these specifically define the *means* to exchange data, not the content
- controlled medical vocabularies (CMVs) such as the Systematized Nomenclature of Medicine, Clinical Terms (SNOMED CT), MEDCIN, Logical Observation Identifiers Names and Codes (LOINC), OpenGALEN Common Reference Model or the highly complex UMLS- used to allow a standard, accurate exchange of data content between systems and providers
- use of hand-held or portable devices to assist providers with data entry/retrieval or medical decision-making, sometimes called mHealth.
- The international standards on the subject are covered by ICS 35.240.80 in which ISO 27799:2008 is one of the core components.
- Molecular bioinformatics and clinical informatics have converged into the field of translational bioinformatics.

History

World wide use of technology in medicine began in the early 1950s with the rise of the computers. In 1949, Gustav Wager established the first professional organization for informatics in Germany. The prehistory, history, and future of medical information and health information technology are discussed in reference. Specialized university departments and Informatics training programs began during the 1960s in France, Germany, Belgium and The Netherlands. Medical informatics research units began to appear during the 1970s in Poland and in the U.S. Since then the development of high-quality health informatics research, education and infrastructure has been the goal of the U.S. and the European Union.

Early names for health informatics included medical computing, medical computer science, computer medicine, medical electronic data processing, medical automatic data processing, medical information processing, medical information science, medical software engineering, and medical computer technology.

Since the 1970s the most prominent international coordinating body has been the International Medical Informatics Association (IMIA).

Medical Informatics in the United States

Even though there was talk about using computers in medicine as technology advanced in the early twentieth century, it was not until the 1950s that informatics really took off in the United States. The earliest use of computation for medicine was for dental projects in the 1950s at the United States National Bureau of Standards by Robert Ledley. The next step in the mid 1950s were the development of expert systems such as MYCIN and Internist-I. In 1965, the National Library of Medicine started to use MEDLINE and MEDLARS. At this time, Neil Pappalardo, Curtis Marble, and Robert Greenes developed MUMPS (Massachusetts General Hospital Utility Multi-Programming System) in Octo Barnett's Laboratory of Computer Science at Massachusetts General Hospital in Boston.

In the 1970s and 1980s it was the most commonly used programming language for clinical applications. The MUMPS operating system was used to support MUMPS language specifications. As of 2004, a descendent of this system is being used in the United States Veterans Affairs hospital system. The VA has the largest enterprise-wide health information system that includes an electronic medical record, known as the Veterans Health Information Systems and Technology Architecture (VistA). A graphical user interface known as the Computerized Patient Record System (CPRS) allows health care providers to review and update a patient's electronic medical record at any of the VA's over 1,000 health care facilities.

In the 1970s a growing number of commercial vendors began to market practice management and electronic medical records systems. Although many products exist, only a small number of health practitioners use fully featured electronic health care records systems.

Homer R. Warner, one of the fathers of medical informatics, founded the Department of Medical Informatics at the University of Utah in 1968. The American Medical Informatics Association (AMIA) has an award named after him on application of informatics to medicine.

Current State of Health Informatics and Policy Initiatives

Americas

Argentina

Since 1997, the Buenos Aires Biomedical Informatics Group, a nonprofit group, represents the interests of a broad range of clinical and non-clinical professionals working within the Health Informatics sphere. Its purposes are:

- Promote the implementation of the computer tool in the healthcare activity, scientific research, health administration and in all areas related to health sciences and biomedical research.

- Support, promote and disseminate content related activities with the management of health information and tools they used to do under the name of Biomedical informatics.

- Promote cooperation and exchange of actions generated in the field of biomedical informatics, both in the public and private, national and international level.

- Interact with all scientists, recognized academic stimulating the creation of new instances that have the same goal and be inspired by the same purpose.

- To promote, organize, sponsor and participate in events and activities for training in computer and information and disseminating developments in this area that might be useful for team members and health related activities.

The Argentinian health system is very heterogeneous, because of that the informatics developments shows an heterogeneous stage. Lot of private Health Care centre has develop system, as the German Hospital of Buenos Aires who was one of the first in develop the electronic health records system.

Brazil

The first applications of computers to medicine and healthcare in Brazil started around 1968, with the installation of the first mainframes in public university hospitals, and the use of programmable calculators in scientific research applications.

Minicomputers, such as the IBM 1130 were installed in several universities, and the first applications were developed for them, such as the hospital census in the School of Medicine of Ribeirão Preto and patient master files, in the Hospital das Clínicas da Universidade de Sao Paulo, respectively at the cities of Ribeirao Preto and Sao Paulo campi of the University of Sao Paulo. In the 1970s, several Digital Corporation and Hewlett Packard minicomputers were acquired for public and Armed Forces hospitals, and more intensively used for intensive-care unit, cardiology diagnostics, patient monitoring and other applications. In the early 1980s, with the arrival of cheaper microcomputers, a great upsurge of computer applications in health ensued, and in 1986 the Brazilian Society of Health Informatics was founded, the first Brazilian Congress of Health Informatics was held, and the first *Brazilian Journal of Health Informatics* was published.

Canada

Health Informatics projects in Canada are implemented provincially, with different provinces creating different systems. A national, federally-funded, not-for-profit organization called Canada Health Infoway was created in 2001 to foster the development and adoption of electronic health records across Canada. As of December 31, 2008 there were 276 EHR projects under way in Canadian hospitals, other health-care facilities, pharmacies and laboratories, with an investment value of $1.5-billion from Canada Health Infoway.

Provincial and territorial programmes include the following:

- eHealth Ontario was created as an Ontario provincial government agency in September 2008. It has been plagued by delays and its CEO was fired over a multimillion-dollar contracts scandal in 2009.
- Alberta Netcare was created in 2003 by the Government of Alberta. Today the netCARE portal is used daily by thousands

of clinicians. It provides access to demographic data, prescribed/ dispensed drugs, known allergies/intolerances, immunizations, laboratory test results, diagnostic imaging reports, the diabetes registry and other medical reports. netCARE interface capabilities are being included in electronic medical record products which are being funded by the provincial government.

United States

In 2004 the U.S. Department of Health and Human Services (HHS) formed the Office of the National Coordinator for Health Information Technology (ONCHIT). The mission of this office is widespread adoption of interoperable electronic health records (EHRs) in the US within 10 years.

The Certification Commission for Healthcare Information Technology (CCHIT), a private nonprofit group, was funded in 2005 by the U.S. Department of Health and Human Services to develop a set of standards for electronic health records (EHR) and supporting networks, and certify vendors who meet them. In July, 2006 CCHIT released its first list of 22 certified ambulatory EHR products, in two different announcements.

Europe

The European Union's Member States are committed to sharing their best practices and experiences to create a European eHealth Area, thereby improving access to and quality health care at the same time as stimulating growth in a promising new industrial sector. The European eHealth Action Plan plays a fundamental role in the European Union's strategy. Work on this initiative involves a collaborative approach among several parts of the Commission services. The European Institute for Health Records is involved in the promotion of high quality electronic health record systems in the European Union.

The NHS in England has contracted out to several vendors for a National Medical Informatics system 'NPFIT' that divides the country into five regions and is to be united by a central electronic medical record system nicknamed "the spine". The project, in 2010, is seriously behind schedule and its scope and design are being revised in real time. The degree of computerisation in NHS secondary was quite high before NPfIT and that programme has had the unfortunate effect of largely stalling further development of the installed base. Almost all general practices in England and Wales are computerised and patients have relatively extensive computerised primary care clinical records. Computerisation is the responsibility of individual practices and there is no single, standardised GP system. Interoperation between primary and secondary care systems is rather primitive.

Scotland has an approach to central connection under way which is more advanced than the English one in some ways. Scotland has the GPASS system whose source code is owned by the State, and controlled and developed by NHS Scotland. It has been provided free to all GPs in Scotland but has developed poorly. Discussion of open sourcing it as a remedy is occurring.

The European Commission's preference, as exemplified in the 5th Framework as well as currently pursued pilot projects, is for Free/ Libre and Open Source Software (FLOSS) for healthcare.

Asia and Oceania

In Asia and Australia-New Zealand, the regional group called the Asia Pacific Association for Medical Informatics (APAMI) was established in 1994 and now consists of more than 15 member regions in the Asia Pacific Region.

Australia

The Australasian College of Health Informatics (ACHI) is the professional association for health informatics in the Asia-Pacific region. It represents the interests of a broad range of clinical and non-clinical professionals working within the health informatics sphere through a commitment to quality, standards and ethical practice. Founded in 2002, ACHI is increasingly valued for its thought leadership, its trusted advisors and national and international experts in Health Informatics. ACHI is an academic institutional member of the International Medical Informatics Association (IMIA) and a full member of the Australian Council of Professions. ACHI is a sponsor of the "e-Journal for Health Informatics", an indexed and peer-reviewed professional journal. ACHI has also supported the "Australian Health Informatics Education Council" (AHIEC) since its founding in 2009.

Although there are a number of health informatics organisations in Australia, the Health Informatics Society of Australia (HISA) is regarded as the major umbrella group and is a member of the International Medical Informatics Association (IMIA). Nursing informaticians were the driving force behind the formation of HISA, which is now a company limited by guarantee of the members. The membership comes from across the informatics spectrum that is from students to corporate affiliates. HISA has a number of branches (Queensland, New South Wales, Victoria and Western Australia) as well as special interest groups such as nursing (NIA), pathology, aged and community care, industry and medical imaging (Conrick, 2006).

Hong Kong

In Hong Kong a computerized patient record system called the Clinical Management System (CMS) has been developed by the Hospital Authority since 1994. This system has been deployed at all the sites of the Authority (40 hospitals and 120 clinics), and is used by all 30,000 clinical staff on a daily basis, with a daily transaction of up to 2 millions. The comprehensive records of 7 million patients are available on-line in the Electronic Patient Record (ePR), with data integrated from all sites. Since 2004 radiology image viewing has been added to the ePR, with radiography images from any HA site being available as part of the ePR.

The Hong Kong Hospital Authority placed particular attention to the governance of clinical systems development, with input from hundreds of clinicians being incorporated through a structured process.

The Health Informatics Section in Hong Kong Hospital Authority has close relationship with Information Technology Department and clinicians to develop healthcare systems for the organization to support the service to all public hospitals and clinics in the region.

The Hong Kong Society of Medical Informatics (HKSMI) was established in 1987 to promote the use of information technology in healthcare. The eHealth Consortium has been formed to bring together clinicians from both the private and public sectors, medical informatics professionals and the IT industry to further promote IT in healthcare in Hong Kong.

India

Religare Technova IT solutions is attempting a new service to improve the healthcare information system in India.

New Zealand

Health Informatics is taught at four New Zealand universities. The most mature and established is the Otago programme which has been offered for over a decade.

Saudi Arabia

The Saudi Association for Health Information (SAHI) was established in 2006 to work under direct supervision of King Saud University for Health Sciences to practice public activities, develop theoretical and applicable knowledge, and provide scientific and applicable studies.

Health Informatics Law

Health informatics law deals with evolving and sometimes complex legal principles as they apply to information technology in health-related fields. It addresses the privacy, ethical and operational issues that invariably arise when electronic tools, information and media are used in health care delivery. Health Informatics Law also applies to all matters that involve information technology, health care and the interaction of information. It deals with the circumstances under which data and records are shared with other fields or areas that support and enhance patient care.

Clinical Informatics

Clinical Informatics is concerned with use information in health care by clinicians.

Clinical informaticians transform health care by analysing, designing, implementing, and evaluating information and communication systems that enhance individual and population health outcomes, improve [patient] care, and strengthen the clinician-patient relationship. Clinical informaticians use their knowledge of patient care combined with their understanding of informatics concepts, methods, and health informatics tools to:

- assess information and knowledge needs of health care professionals and patients,
- characterize, evaluate, and refine clinical processes,
- develop, implement, and refine clinical decision support systems, and
- lead or participate in the procurement, customization, development, implementation, management, evaluation, and continuous improvement of clinical information systems.

Physicians who are board-certified in clinical informatics collaborate with other health care and information technology professionals to develop health informatics tools which promote patient care that is safe, efficient, effective, timely, patient-centered, and equitable.

Translational Bioinformatics

With the completion of the human genome and the recent advent of high throughput sequencing and genome-wise association studies of single nucleotide polymorphisms, the fields of molecular bioinformatics, biostatistiques, statistical genetics and clinical informatics are converging into the emerging field of translational bioinformatics.

DNA Sequencing Theory

DNA sequencing theory is the broad body of work that attempts to lay analytical foundations for DNA sequencing. The practical aspects revolve around designing and optimizing sequencing projects, predicting project performance, troubleshooting experimental results, characterizing factors such as sequence bias and the effects of software processing algorithms, and comparing various sequencing methods to one another. In this sense, it could be considered a branch of systems engineering or operations research. The permanent archive of work is primarily mathematical, although numerical calculations are often conducted for particular problems too. DNA sequencing theory addresses *physical processes* related to sequencing DNA and should not be confused with theories of analysing resultant DNA sequences, e.g. sequence alignment. Publications sometimes do not make a careful distinction, but the latter are primarily concerned with algorithmic issues.

Sequencing as a Covering Problem

All mainstream methods of DNA sequencing rely on reading small fragments of DNA and subsequently reconstructing these data to infer the original DNA target, either via assembly or alignment to a reference. The abstraction common to these methods is that of a mathematical covering problem. For example, one can imagine a line segment representing the target and a subsequent process where smaller segments are "dropped" onto random locations of the target. The target is considered "sequenced" when adequate coverage accumulates, for example when no gaps remain.

The abstract properties of covering have been studied by mathematicians for over a century. However, direct application of these results has not generally been possible. Closed-form mathematical solutions, especially for probability distributions, often cannot be readily evaluated. That is, they involve inordinately large amounts of computer time for parameters characteristic of DNA sequencing. Stevens' configuration is one such example. Results obtained from the perspective of pure mathematics also do not account for factors that are actually important in sequencing, for instance detectable overlap in sequencing fragments, double-stranding, edge-effects, and target multiplicity. Consequently, development of sequencing theory has proceeded more according to the philosophy of applied mathematics. In particular, it has been problem-focused and makes expedient use of approximations, simulations, etc.

Lander-Waterman Theory

In 1988, Eric Lander and Michael Waterman published an important paper examining the covering problem from the standpoint of gaps. Although they focused on the so-called mapping problem, the abstraction to sequencing is much the same. They furnished a number of useful results that were adopted as the standard theory from the earliest days of "large-scale" genome sequencing. Their model was also used in designing the Human Genome Project and continues to play an important role in DNA sequencing.

Ultimately, the main goal of a sequencing project is to close all gaps, so the "gap perspective" was a logical basis of developing a sequencing model. One of the more frequently used results from this model is the expected number of contigs, given the number of fragments sequenced. If one neglects the amount of sequence that is essentially "wasted" by having to detect overlaps, their theory yields.

$$E\langle \text{contigs} \rangle = Ne^{-R}.$$

In 1995, Roach proposed a model that appeared to be essentially different and asserted that Lander-Waterman theory gave contradictory results for large values of R. Wendl and Waterston later showed, based on Stevens' method, that subtle differences in interpretation explained the anomalies and that both models were indeed essentially identical and consistent.

The basic ideas of Lander-Waterman theory led to a number of additional results for particular variations in mapping techniques. However, technological advancements have rendered mapping and its more esoteric theories largely obsolete.

Recent Advancements

The physical processes and protocols of DNA sequencing have continued to evolve, largely driven by advancements in bio-chemical methods, hardware, and automation techniques. There is now a wide range of problems that DNA sequencing has made in-roads into, including metagenomics and medical (cancer) sequencing.

There are important factors in these scenarios that classical theory does not account for. Recent work has begun to focus on resolving the effects of some of these issues. The level of mathematics becomes commensurately more sophisticated.

Multiplicity

Biologists have developed methods to filter highly-repetitive, essentially un-sequenceable regions of genomes. These procedures are important for organisms whose genomes consist mostly of such DNA, for example corn. They yield multitudes of small islands of sequenceable DNA products. Wendl and Barbazuk proposed an extension to Lander-Waterman Theory to account for "gaps" in the target due to filtering and the so-called "edge-effect". The latter is a position-specific sampling bias, for example the terminal base position has only a $1/G$ chance of being covered, as opposed to L/G for interior positions. For $R < 1$, classical Lander-Waterman Theory still gives good predictions, but dynamics change for higher redundancies.

Paired-end Sequencing

Modern sequencing methods usually sequence both ends of a larger fragment, which provides linking information for *de novo* assembly and improved probabilities for alignment to reference sequence. Researchers generally believe that longer lengths of data (read lengths) enhance performance for very large DNA targets, an idea consistent with predictions from distribution models. However, Wendl showed that smaller fragments provide better coverage on small, linear targets because they reduce the edge effect in linear molecules. These findings have implications for sequencing the products of DNA filtering procedures. Read-pairing and fragment size evidently have negligible influence for large, whole-genome class targets.

Diploid Sequencing

Sequencing is emerging as an important tool in medicine, for example in cancer research. Here, the ability to detect heterozygous mutations is important and this can only be done if the sequence of the diploid genome is obtained. In the pioneering efforts to sequence individuals, Levy *et al.* and Wheeler *et al.*, who sequenced Craig Venter and Jim Watson, respectively, outlined models for covering both alleles in a genome. Wendl and Wilson followed with a more general theory that allowed for an arbitrary number of coverings of each allele and arbitrary ploidy. These results point to the general conclusion that the amount of data needed for such projects is significantly higher than for traditional haploid projects.

Limitations

DNA sequencing theories often invoke the assumption that certain random variables in a model are independently and identically distributed. For example, in Lander-Waterman Theory, a sequenced fragment is presumed to have the same probability of covering each region of a genome and all fragments are assumed to be independent of one another.

In actuality, sequencing projects are subject to various types of bias, including differences of how well regions can be cloned, sequencing anomalies, biases in the target sequence (which is *not* random), and software-dependent errors and biases.

In general, theory will agree well with observation up to the point that enough data have been generated to expose latent biases. The kinds of biases related to the underlying target sequence are particularly difficult to model, since the sequence itself may not be known *a priori*. This presents a type of "chicken and egg" closure problem.

Academic Status

Sequencing theory is based on elements of mathematics, biology, and systems engineering, so it is highly interdisciplinary. Although many universities now have programs in computational biology, there does not yet seem to be a strong focus at the graduate level on this topic. Academic contributions have mainly been limited to a small number of PhD dissertations.

Dot Plot (Bioinformatics)

A dot plot (aka contact plot or residue contact map) is a graphical method that allows the comparison of two biological sequences and identify regions of close similarity between them. It is a kind of recurrence plot.

Introduction

The simplest way to visualize the similarity between two protein sequences is to use a similarity matrix, known as a dot plot. These were introduced by Philips in the 1970s and are two-dimensional matrices which have the sequences of the proteins being compared along the vertical and horizontal axes. For a simple visual representation of the similarity between two sequences, individual cells in the matrix can be shaded black if residues are identical, so that matching sequence segments appear as runs of diagonal lines across the matrix.

Some idea of the similarity of the two sequences can be gleaned from the number and length of matching segments shown in the matrix. Identical proteins will obviously have a diagonal line in the centre of the matrix. Insertions and deletions between sequences give rise to disruptions in this diagonal. Regions of local similarity or repetitive sequences give rise to further diagonal matches in addition to the central diagonal. Because of the limited protein alphabet, many matching sequence segments may simply have arisen by chance. One way of reducing this noise is to only shade runs or 'tuples' of residues, e.g. a tuple of 3 corresponds to three residues in a row. This is effective because the probability of matching three residues in a row by chance is much lower than single-residue matches.

Dot Plots are one of the oldest ways of comparing two sequences. They compare two sequences by organizing one sequence on the x-axis, and another on the y-axis, of a plot. When the residues of both sequences match at the same location on the plot, a dot is drawn at the corresponding position. Note, that the sequences can be written backwards or forwards, however the sequences on both axes must be written in the same direction.

Also note, that the direction of the sequences on the axes will determine the direction of the line on the dot plot. Once the dots have been plotted, they will combine to form lines. The closeness of the sequences in similarity will determine how close the diagonal line is to what a graph showing a curve demonstrating a direct relationship is. This relationship is affected by certain sequence features such as frame shifts, direct repeats, and inverted repeats. Frame shifts include insertions, deletions, and mutations. The presence of one of these features, or the presence of multiple features, will cause for multiple lines to be plotted in a various possibility of configurations, depending on the features present in the sequences. A feature that will cause a very different result on the dot plot is the presence of low-complexity region/regions. Low-complexity regions are regions in the sequence with only a few amino acids, which in turn, causes redundancy within that small or limited region. These regions are typically found around the diagonal, and may or may not have a square in the middle of the dot plot.

Example

Example of a dot plot for comparing two simple protein sequences:

1. All cells associated with identical residue pairs between the sequences are shaded black;

2. only those cells associated with identical tuples of two residues are shaded black; and

3. only cells associated with tuples of three are shaded and the optimal path through the matrix has been drawn.

This is constrained to be within the window given by the two black lines parallel to the central diagonal. An alternative high-scoring path is also shown.

Functional Genomics

Functional genomics is a field of molecular biology that attempts to make use of the vast wealth of data produced by genomic projects (such as genome sequencing projects) to describe gene (and protein) functions and interactions. Unlike genomics and proteomics, functional genomics focuses on the dynamic aspects such as gene transcription, translation, and protein-protein interactions, as opposed to the static aspects of the genomic information such as DNA sequence or structures. Functional genomics attempts to answer questions about the function of DNA at the levels of genes, RNA transcripts, and protein products. A key characteristic of functional genomics studies is their genome-wide approach to these questions, generally involving high-throughput methods rather than a more traditional "gene-by-gene" approach.

Goals of Functional Genomics

The goal of functional genomics is to understand the relationship between an organism's genome and its phenotype. The term functional genomics is often used broadly to refer to the many possible approaches to understanding the properties and function of the entirety of an organism's genes and gene products. This definition is somewhat variable; Gibson and Muse define it as "approaches under development to ascertain the biochemical, cellular, and/or physiological properties of each and every gene product", while Pevsner includes the study of nongenic elements in his definition: "the genome-wide study of the function of DNA (including genes and nongenic elements), as well as the nucleic acid and protein products encoded by DNA".

Because of its genome-wide approach, functional genomics requires the use of high-throughput technologies capable of assaying many functions or relationships simultaneously. Functional genomics involves studies of natural variation in genes, RNA, and proteins over time (such as an organism's development) or space (such as its body regions), as well as studies of natural or experimental functional disruptions affecting genes, chromosomes, RNAs, or proteins. The promise of functional genomics is to expand and synthesize genomic and proteomic knowledge into an understanding of the dynamic properties of an organism at cellular and/or organismal levels. This would provide a more complete picture of how biological function arises from the information encoded in an organism's genome. The possibility of understanding how a particular mutation leads to a given phenotype has important implications for human genetic diseases, as answering these questions could point scientists in the direction of a treatment or cure.

Techniques and Applications

Functional genomics includes function-related aspects of the genome itself such as mutation and polymorphism (such as SNP) analysis, as well as measurement of molecular activities. The latter comprise a number of "-omics" such as transcriptomics (gene expression), proteomics (protein expression), phosphoproteomics (a subset of proteomics) and metabolomics. Functional genomics uses mostly multiplex techniques to measure the abundance of many or all gene products such as mRNAs or proteins within a biological sample. Together these measurement modalities endeavor to quantitate the various biological processes and improve our understanding of gene and protein functions and interactions.

At the DNA Level

Genetic Interaction Mapping

Systematic pairwise deletion of genes or inhibition of gene expression can be used to identify genes with related function, even if they do not interact physically. Epistasis refers to the fact that effects for two different gene knockouts may not be additive; that is, the phenotype that results when two genes are inhibited may be different from the sum of the effects of single knockouts.

The ENCODE Project

The ENCODE (Encyclopedia of DNA elements) project is an in-depth analysis of the human genome whose goal is to identify all the functional elements of genomic DNA, in both coding and noncoding regions. To this point, only the pilot phase of the study has been completed, involving hundreds of assays performed on 44 regions of known or unknown function comprising 1% of the human genome. Important results include evidence from genomic tiling arrays that most nucleotides are transcribed as coding transcripts, noncoding RNAs, or random transcripts, the discovery of additional transcriptional regulatory sites, further elucidation of chromatin-modifying mechanisms.

At the RNA Level: Transcriptome Profiling

Microarrays

Microarrays measure the amount of mRNA in a sample that corresponds to a given gene or probe DNA sequence. Probe sequences are immobilized on a solid surface and allowed to hybridize with fluorescently-labelled "target" mRNA. The intensity of fluorescence of a spot is proportional to the amount of target sequence that has hybridized to that spot, and therefore to the abundance of that mRNA sequence in the sample. Microarrays allow for identification of candidate genes involved in a given process based on variation between transcript levels for different conditions and shared expression patterns with genes of known function.

SAGE

SAGE (Serial analysis of gene expression) is an alternate method of gene expression analysis based on RNA sequencing rather than hybridization. SAGE relies on the sequencing of 10-17 base pair tags which are unique to each gene. These tags are produced from poly-A mRNA and ligated end-to-end before sequencing. SAGE gives an unbiased measurement of the number of transcripts per cell, since it does not depend on prior knowledge of what transcripts to study (as microarrays do).

At the Protein Level: Protein-protein Interactions

Yeast Two-hybrid System

A yeast two-hybrid (Y2H) screen tests a "bait" protein against many potential interacting proteins ("prey") to identify physical protein-protein interactions. This system is based on a transcription factor, originally GAL4, whose separate DNA-binding and transcription activation domains are both required in order for the protein to cause transcription of a reporter gene.

In a Y2H screen, the "bait" protein is fused to the binding domain of GAL4, and a library of potential "prey" (interacting) proteins is recombinantly expressed in a vector with the activation domain. In vivo interaction of bait and prey proteins in a yeast cell brings the activation and binding domains of GAL4 close enough together to result in expression of a reporter gene. It is also possible to systematically test a library of bait proteins against a library of prey proteins to identify all possible interactions in a cell.

AP/MS

Affinity purification and mass spectrometry (AP/MS) is able to identify proteins that interact with one another in complexes. Complexes of proteins are allowed to form around a particular "bait" protein. The bait protein is identified using an antibody or a recombinant tag which allows it to be extracted along with any proteins that have formed a complex with it. The proteins are then digested into short peptide fragments and mass spectrometry is used to identify the proteins based on the mass-to-charge ratios of those fragments.

Loss-of-function Techniques

Mutagenesis

Gene function can be investigated by systematically "knocking out" genes one by one. This is done by either deletion or disruption of function (such as by insertional mutagenesis) and the resulting organisms are screened for phenotypes that provide clues to the function of the disrupted gene.

RNAi

RNA interference (RNAi) methods can be used to transiently silence or knock down gene expression using ~20 base-pair double-stranded RNA typically delivered by transfection of synthetic ~20-mer short-interfering RNA molecules (siRNAs) or by virally-encoded short-hairpin RNAs (shRNAs). RNAi screens, typically performed in cell culture-based assays or experimental organisms (such as C. elegans) can be used to systematically disrupt nearly every gene in a genome or subsets of genes (sub-genomes); possible functions of disrupted genes can be assigned based on observed phenotypes.

Functional Annotations for Genes

Genome Annotation

Putative genes can be identified by scanning a genome for regions likely to encode proteins, based on characteristics such as long open reading frames, transcriptional initiation sequences, and polyadenylation sites. A sequence identified as a putative gene must be confirmed by further evidence, such as similarity to cDNA or EST sequences from the same organism, similarity of the predicted protein sequence to known proteins, association with promoter sequences, or evidence that mutating the sequence produces an observable phenotype.

Rosetta Stone Approach

The Rosetta stone approach is a computation method of de novo protein function prediction, based on the hypothesis that some proteins involved in a given physiological process may exist as two separate genes in one organism and as a single gene in another. Genomes are scanned for sequences that are independent in one organism and in a single open reading frame in another. If two genes have fused, it is predicted that they have similar biological functions that make such coregulation advantageous.

Functional Genomics and Bioinformatics

Because of the large quantity of data produced by these techniques and the desire to find biologically meaningful patterns, bioinformatics is crucial to analysis of functional genomics data. Examples of techniques in this class are data clustering or principal component analysis for unsupervised machine learning (class detection) as well as artificial neural networks or support vector machines for supervised machine learning (class prediction, classification).

Margaret Oakley Dayhoff

Dr. Margaret Belle (Oakley) Dayhoff (March 11, 1925 – 1983) was an American physical chemist and a pioneer in the field of bioinformatics. Dr. Dayhoff was a professor at Georgetown University Medical Centre and a noted research biochemist at the National Biomedical Research Foundation where she pioneered the application of mathematics and computational methods to the field of biochemistry. She dedicated her career to applying the evolving computational technologies to support advances in biology and medicine, most notably the creation of protein and nucleic acid databases and tools to interrogate the databases. Her PhD degree was from Columbia University in the Department of Chemistry, where she devised computational methods to calculate molecular resonance energies of several organic compounds. She did postdoctoral studies at the Rockefeller Institute (now Rockefeller University) and the University of Maryland, and joined the newly established National Biomedical Research Foundation in 1959. She was the first woman to hold office in the Biophysical Society, first as Secretary and eventually President. She originated one of the first substitution matrices, Point accepted mutations (*PAM*). The one-letter code used for amino acids was developed by her, reflecting an attempt to reduce the size of the data files used to describe amino acid sequences in an era of punch-card computing.

Early Life

Dayhoff was born an only child in Philadelphia, but moved to New York City as a child. Her academic promise was evident from the outset; she was valedictorian (class of 1942) at Bayside High School, Bayside, New York and from there received a scholarship to Washington Square College of New York University, graduating magna cum laude in mathematics in 1945.

Research

From there, Dayhoff undertook a Ph.D. in quantum chemistry, under George Kimball, in the Columbia University Department of Chemistry. In her graduate thesis, Dayhoff had pioneered the use of computer capabilities — i.e., mass-data processing — to theoretical chemistry; specifically, she applied punch card machines to calculate the resonance energies of several polycyclic organic molecules.

After completing her Ph.D, Dayhoff studied electrochemistry at the Rockefeller Institute from 1948 to 1951. In 1952, she moved to Maryland with her family and later received a research fellowship from the University of Maryland (1957–1959), working on a model of chemical bonding with Ellis Lippincott. She taught physiology and biophysics for 13 years, while becoming affiliated with the National Biomedical Research Foundation, a Fellow of the American Association for the Advancement of Science, a councillor of the International Society for the Study of the Origins of Life (1980) and acting on the editorial boards of DNA, Journal of Molecular Evolution and Computers in Biology and Medicine.

Frederic Sanger's determination of the first complete amino acid sequence of a protein (insulin) in 1955, led a number of researchers to sequence various proteins from different species. In the early 1960s, a theory was developed that small differences between homologous protein sequences (sequences with a high likelihood of common ancestry) could indicate the process and rate of evolutionary change on the molecular level. The notion that such molecular analysis could help scientists decode evolutionary patterns in organisms was formalized in the published papers of Emile Zuckerkandl and Linus Pauling in 1962 and 1965. Dayhoff worked side by side with Lippincott and Carl Sagan on thermodynamic models of cosmo-chemical systems, including prebiological planetary atmospheres.

Dayhoff went on to pioneer the development of programmable computer methods for use in comparing protein sequences and deriving their evolutionary histories (in other words, discerning homologies) from their sequence alignments. Though this was before the days of massive outputs of sequence information by automated and other methods, Margaret Dayhoff anticipated the potential of computers to the current theories of Zuckerkandl & Pauling and the method which Sanger had engineered.

With Richard Eck, she published the first reconstruction of a phylogeny (evolutionary tree) by computers from molecular sequences, using a maximum parsimony method. She also formulated the first probability model of protein evolution, the PAM model, in 1966.

She initiated the collection of protein sequences in the Atlas of Protein Sequence and Structure, a book collecting all known protein sequences that she published in 1965. It was subsequently republished in several editions. This led to the Protein Information Resource database of protein sequences, which was developed by her group. It and the parallel effort by Walter Goad which led to the GenBank database of nucleic acid sequences are the twin origins of the modern databases of molecular sequences. The Atlas was organized by gene families, and she is regarded as a pioneer in their recognition. Her approach to proteins was always determinedly evolutionary. Margaret Oakley Dayoff died of a heart attack at the age of 57.

David Lipman has called Dayhoff the mother and father of bioinformatics. Lipman, who is director of the National Centre for Biotechnology Information is also the scientist who spearheaded the collaborative project that produced BLAST. His ongoing work in developing better computational methods for molecular biology attests to his inheritance of Dayhoff's legacy.

Metabolic Network Modelling

Metabolic network reconstruction and simulation allows for an in depth insight into comprehending the molecular mechanisms of a particular organism, especially correlating the genome with molecular physiology (Francke, Siezen, and Teusink 2005). A reconstruction breaks down metabolic pathways into their respective reactions and enzymes, and analyses them within the perspective of the entire network. Examples of various metabolic pathways include glycolysis, Krebs cycle, pentose phosphate pathway. In simplified terms, a reconstruction involves collecting all of the relevant metabolic information of an organism and then compiling it in a way that makes sense for various types of analyses to be performed. The correlation between the genome and metabolism is made by searching gene databases, such as KEGG, GeneDB, for particular genes by inputting enzyme or protein names. For example, a search can be conducted based on the protein name or the EC number (a number that represents the catalytic function of the enzyme of interest) in order to find the associated gene.

Beginning Steps of a Reconstruction

Resources

Below is more detailed description of a few gene/enzyme/reaction/ pathway databases that are crucial to a metabolic reconstruction:

- Kyoto Encyclopedia of Genes and Genomes (KEGG): This is a bioinformatics database containing information on genes, proteins, reactions, and pathways. The 'KEGG Organisms' section, which is divided into eukaryotes and prokaryotes, encompasses many organisms for which gene and DNA information can be searched by typing in the enzyme of choice.

This resource can be extremely useful when building the association between metabolism enzymes, reactions and genes.

- BioCyc, EcoCyc, and MetaCyc: BioCyc is a collection of 1,000 pathway/genome databases (as of Oct 2010), with each database dedicated to one organism. For example, EcoCyc is a highly detailed bioinformatics database on the genome and metabolic reconstruction of *Escherichia Coli*, including thorough descriptions of *E. coli* signalling pathways and regulatory network. The EcoCyc database can serve as a paradigm and model for any reconstruction. Additionally, MetaCyc, an encyclopedia of experimentally defined metabolic pathways and enzymes, contains 1,500 metabolic pathways and 8,700 metabolic reactions (Oct 2010).

- Pathway Tools: A bioinformatics software package that assists in the construction of pathway/genome databases such as EcoCyc (Karp 2010). Developed by Peter Karp and associates at the SRI International Bioinformatics Group, Pathway Tools comprises several separate units. First, PathoLogic takes an annotated genome for an organism and infers probable metabolic pathways to produce a new pathway/genome database. This can be followed by application of the Pathway Hole Filler, which predicts likely genes to fill "holes" (missing steps) in predicted pathways. Afterward, the Pathway Tools Navigator and Editor functions let users visualize, analyse, access and update the database. Thus, using PathoLogic and encyclopedias like MetaCyc, an initial fast reconstruction can be developed automatically, and then using the other units of Pathway Tools, a very detailed manual update, curation and verification step can be carried out (SRI 2005).

- ERGO: ERGO integrates data from every level including genomic, biochemical data, literature, and high-throughput analysis into a comprehensive user friendly network of metabolic and nonmetabolic pathways.

- metaTIGER: is a collection of metabolic profiles and phylogenomic information on a taxonomically diverse range of eukaryotes. Phylogenomic information is provided by 2,257 large phylogenetic trees which can be interactively explored. High-throughput tree analysis can also be carried out to identify trees of interest, e.g. trees containing horizontal gene transfers.

metaTIGER also provides novel facilities for viewing and comparing the metabolic profiles.

- ENZYME: This is an enzyme nomenclature database (part of the ExPASY proteonomics server of the Swiss Institute of Bioinformatics). After searching for a particular enzyme on the database, this resource gives you the reaction that is catalysed. Additionally, ENZYME has direct links to various other gene/enzyme/medical literature databases such as KEGG, BRENDA, PUBMED, and PUMA2 to name a few.

- BRENDA: A comprehensive enzyme database, BRENDA, allows you to search for an enzyme by name or EC number. You can also search for an organism and find all the relevant enzyme information. Moreover, when an enzyme search is carried out, BRENDA provides a list of all organisms containing the particular enzyme of interest.

- PUBMED: This is an online library developed by the National Centre for Biotechnology Information, which contains a massive collection of medical journals. Using the link provided by ENZYME, the search can be directed towards the organism of interest, thus recovering literature on the enzyme and its use inside of the organism.

Next Steps of the Reconstruction

After the initial stages of the reconstruction, a systematic verification is made in order to make sure no inconsistencies are present and that all the entries listed are correct and accurate (Francke et al. 2005). Furthermore, previous literature can be researched in order to support any information obtained from one of the many metabolic reaction and genome databases. This provides an added level of assurance for the reconstruction that the enzyme and the reaction it catalyses do actually occur in the organism.

Any new reactions not present in the databases need to be added to the reconstruction. The presence or absence of certain reactions of the metabolism will affect the amount of reactants/products that are present for other reactions within the particular pathway. This is because products in one reaction go on to become the reactants for another reaction, i.e. products of one reaction can combine with other proteins or compounds to form new proteins/compounds in the presence of different enzymes or catalysts.

Francke *et al.* (2005) provide an excellent example as to why the verification step of the project needs to be performed in significant detail. During a metabolic network reconstruction of *Lactobacillus plantarum*, the model showed that succinyl-CoA was one of the reactants for a reaction that was a part of the biosynthesis of methionine. However, an understanding of the physiology of the organism would have revealed that due to an incomplete tricarboxylic acid pathway, *Lactobacillus plantarum* does not actually produce succinyl-CoA, and the correct reactant for that part of the reaction was acetyl-CoA.

Therefore, systematic verification of the initial reconstruction will bring to light several inconsistencies that can adversely affect the final interpretation of the reconstruction, which is to accurately comprehend the molecular mechanisms of the organism. Furthermore, the simulation step also ensures that all the reactions present in the reconstruction are properly balanced. To sum up, a reconstruction that is fully accurate can lead to greater insight about understanding the functioning of the organism of interest.

Advantages of a Reconstruction

- Several inconsistencies exist between gene, enzyme, and reaction databases and published literature sources regarding the metabolic information of an organism. A reconstruction is a systematic verification and compilation of data from various sources that takes into account all of the discrepancies.
- A reconstruction combines the relevant metabolic and genomic information of an organism.
- A reconstruction also allows for metabolic comparisons to be performed between various species of the same organism as well as between different organisms.

Metabolic Network Simulation

A metabolic network can be broken down into a stoichiometric matrix where the rows represent the compounds of the reactions, while the columns of the matrix correspond to the reactions themselves. Stoichiometry is a quantitative relationship between substrates of a chemical reaction (Merriam 2002). In order to deduce what the metabolic network suggests, recent research has centered on two approaches; namely extreme pathways and elementary mode analysis.

Extreme Pathways

Price, Reed, Papin, Wiback and Palsson (2003) use a method of singular value decomposition (SVD) of extreme pathways in order to understand regulation of a human red blood cell metabolism. Extreme pathways are convex basis vectors that consist of steady state functions of a metabolic network. For any particular metabolic network, there is always a unique set of extreme pathways available (Papin *et al.* 2004). Furthermore, Price *et al.* (2003) define a constraint-based approach, where through the help of constraints like mass balance and maximum reaction rates, it is possible to develop a 'solution space' where all the feasible options fall within. Then, using a kinetic model approach, a single solution that falls within the extreme pathway solution space can be determined (Price *et al.* 2003). Therefore, in their study, Price *et al.* (2003) use both constraint and kinetic approaches to understand the human red blood cell metabolism. In conclusion, using extreme pathways, the regulatory mechanisms of a metabolic network can be studied in further detail.

Elementary Mode Analysis

Elementary mode analysis closely matches the approach used by extreme pathways. Similar to extreme pathways, there is always a unique set of elementary modes available for a particular metabolic network (Papin *et al.* 2004). These are the smallest sub-networks that allow a metabolic reconstruction network to function in steady state. According to Stelling *et al.* (2002), elementary modes can be used to understand cellular objectives for the overall metabolic network. Furthermore, elementary mode analysis takes into account stoichiometrics and thermodynamics when evaluating whether a particular metabolic route or network is feasible and likely for a set of proteins/enzymes.

Minimal Metabolic Behaviours (MMBs)

Recently, Larhlimi and Bockmayr (2009) presented a new approach called "minimal metabolic Behaviours" for the analysis of metabolic networks. Like elementary modes or extreme pathways, these are uniquely determined by the network, and yield a complete description of the flux cone. However, the new description is much more compact. In contrast with elementary modes and extreme pathways, which use an inner description based on generating vectors of the flux cone, MMBs are using an outer description of the flux cone. This approach is based on sets of non-negativity constraints. These can be identified with irreversible reactions, and thus have a direct biochemical interpretation. One can characterize a metabolic network by MMBs and the reversible metabolic space.

Flux Balance Analysis

A different technique to simulate the metabolic network is to perform flux balance analysis. This method uses linear programming, but in contrast to elementary mode analysis and extreme pathways, only a single solution results in the end. Linear programming is usually used to obtain the maximum potential of the objective function that you are looking at, and therefore, when using flux balance analysis, a single solution is found to the optimization problem. In a flux balance analysis approach, exchange fluxes are assigned to those metabolites that enter or leave the particular network only. Those metabolites that are consumed within the network are not assigned any exchange flux value. Also, the exchange fluxes along with the enzymes can have constraints ranging from a negative to positive value (ex: -10 to 10).

Furthermore, this particular approach can accurately define if the reaction stoichiometry is in line with predictions by providing fluxes for the balanced reactions. Also, flux balance analysis can highlight the most effective and efficient pathway through the network in order to achieve a particular objective function. In addition, gene knockout studies can be performed using flux balance analysis. The enzyme that correlates to the gene that needs to be removed is given a constraint value of 0. Then, the reaction that the particular enzyme catalyses is completely removed from the analysis.

Dynamic Simulation and Parameter Estimation

In order to perform a dynamic simulation with such a network it is necessary to construct an ordinary differential equation system that describes the rates of change in each metabolite's concentration or amount. To this end, a rate law, i.e., a kinetic equation is required for each reaction. Often these rate laws contain kinetic parameters with uncertain values. In many cases it is desired to estimate these parameter values with respect to given time-series data of metabolite concentrations. The system is then supposed to reproduce the given data. For this purpose the distance between the given data set and the result of the simulation, i.e., the numerically or in few cases analytically obtained solution of the differential equation system is computed. The values of the parameters are then estimated to minimize this distance. One step further, it may be desired to estimate the mathematical structure of the differential equation system because the real rate laws are not known for the reactions within the system under study. To this end, the program SBMLsqueezer allows automatic creation of appropriate rate laws for all reactions with the network.

Molecular Design Software

Molecular design software is a software for molecular modelling, distinctive property of which is the presence of the special support for developing the molecular models.

In contrast to the usual molecular modelling programs such as the molecular dynamics and quantum chemistry programs, such software directly supports the aspects related to the construction of molecular models:

- Molecular graphics
- interactive molecular drawing and conformational editing
- building of polymeric molecules, crystals and solvated systems
- partial charges development
- geometry optimization
- support for the different aspects of Force Field development, *etc.*

Molecular Modelling on GPU

Molecular modelling on GPU is the technique of using a graphics processing unit (GPU) for molecular simulations.

In 2007, NVIDIA introduced video cards that could be used not only to show graphics but also for scientific calculations. These cards include many arithmetic units (currently up to 240) working in parallel. Long before this event, the computational power of video cards was used to accelerate calculations. What was new is that stream processing made it possible to develop parallel programs in a high-level language. This technology substantially simplified programming by enabling programs to be written in C/C++.

Quantum chemistry calculations and molecular mechanics simulations (molecular modelling in terms of classical mechanics) are among beneficial applications of this technology. The video cards can accelerate the calculations tens of times. Thus, a PC with such a card has the power similar to that of a cluster of workstations based on the common processors.

Morphometrics

Morphometrics is a field concerned with studying variation and change in the form (size and shape) of organisms or objects. There are several methods for extracting data from shapes, each with their own benefits and weaknesses. These include measurement of lengths and angles, landmark analysis and outline analysis.

Morphometric analyses are commonly performed on organisms, and are particularly useful in analysing the fossil record. In this use, it is assumed that morphometrics can quantify a trait of evolutionary significance, and by detecting changes in the shape of organisms, deduce something of their ontogeny or evolutionary relationships. "Morphometrics", in the broader sense of the term, is also used to precisely locate certain areas of featureless organs such as the brain, and is used in describing the shape of other things.

Advantages of Morphometrics

Morphometrics adds a quantitative element to descriptions, allowing more rigorous comparisons. It enables one to describe complex shapes in a rigorous fashion, and permits numerical comparison between different forms. By reducing shape to a series of numbers, it allows objective comparison that does not rely on individuals' interpretation of descriptive words. Further, statistical analysis can highlight areas where change is concentrated, removing the need to explicitly declare an area for investigation before study.

Forms of Morphometrics

Morphometric study aims to describe the shape of an object in the simplest possible fashion, removing extraneous information and thereby facilitating comparison between different objects.

An object's shape be described in many ways – one may take a sequence of defined measurements, record the position of certain important landmarks, or define the outline of the object. Each of these exaggerates a certain aspect of an object. Morphometric analysis begins by obtaining and (usually) digitising one of these suites of descriptors. Since morphometrics is concerned solely with shape, analysis begins by removing confounding factors – size, rotation and location must all be corrected for.

Typically, analysis begins with principal component analysis, which highlights any trends and makes it easy to spot any correlation with other features.

"Traditional" Morphometrics

The traditional, and most rudimentary, method of morphometrics involves measuring distances, angles and areas. Commonly, the measurements taken are of little significance in terms of the organism. The method has the drawback that many measurements covary, thwarting statistical analysis – for instance, tibia length will vary with arm length, and the interdependence of these two variables will bias the data set.

The methodology is useful in cases where linear and angular data are available, and is of great utility in study of growth. However, it can only distinguish changes in length, and cannot be used to map how these changes are accomplished.

Geometric Morphometrics

This technique assesses the distribution of "landmarks": points described by a tightly defined set of rules, for example the suture between three named bones in a skull.

Selecting Landmarks

The technique only generates data that are as good as the landmarks that are input, and many studies are called into question as a result of suspect landmark selection. Well chosen landmarks reflect homologous points – i.e. points with evolutionary significance. In order for a landmark to be of utility, it must be present on all specimens studied. The number of landmarks which can provide meaningful data is approximately equal to the number of specimens sampled: if there are more landmarks than specimens, some landmarks are redundant, and results produced may be unsubstantiated.

Types of Landmark

There are three categories of landmarks, listed here in order of decreasing utility. True landmarks represent a genuine homologous structure. Pseudolandmarks are marks defined by relative locations; for example, "the point of highest curvature of this bone." Semilandmarks are defined relative to other landmarks, for example "midway between landmarks X and Y." The latter are of less value and often weighted against in analyses.

Reaching the "Shape"

Removing Translation

In order to compare shapes, they need to be fitted into a frame of reference that places them in the same virtual space. With landmarks, this can be done by lining up one specific landmark; this has the disadvantage that it removes all the data from this point. A preferable (but not error-free) method is to use the centroid – that is, the "centre of mass" of the landmarks, assigning an equal weight to each landmark. This centroid is calculated for each specimen and translated to the origin.

Removing Size Differences

Objects must be scaled to the same relative size. In an ideal world this could be done by adjusting everything to a fixed measure of size, for example based on mass. However, such reliable measures of body size are usually lacking, and as such the spread of the landmarks must be used as a proxy for size. A simple approach is to scale the landmarks such that the distance between two named landmarks is constant in all specimens; however, this removes data from these two landmarks, and has the implicit assumption that the two are an equivalent distance apart in all specimens. A better method has since been developed, which involves calculating the distance of each landmark from the centroid, calculating the square root of the squares of individual distances (the "centroid size"), and setting this to 1 for each specimen.

Removing Rotation

Rotation is the final non-shape attribute that must be removed from datasets prior to their interpretation. This is performed by minimising the sum of squared distances between corresponding landmarks on subsequent specimens.

Superimposition

Various techniques have been developed to perform these three stages in one step. Bookstein registration is simpler on many levels, and was traditionally used, but strips the data from two landmarks. It involves setting two landmarks to the fixed co-ordinates $(0,0)$ and $(0,1)$ to combine the previous steps. Better is Procrustes superimposition, which combines the least squares approaches previously discussed into one algorithm.

Chapter 4

Softwares and their Applications

Clustal. W.

Clustal is a widely used multiple sequence alignment computer program. The latest version is 2.1. There are two main variations:

- ClustalW: command line interface
- ClustalX: This version has a graphical user interface. It is available for Windows, Mac OS, and Unix/Linux.

Input/Output

This program accepts a wide range on input format. Included NBRF/PIR, FASTA, EMBL/Swissprot, Clustal, GCC/MSF, GCG9 RSF, and GDE.

The output format can be one or many of the following: Clustal, NBRF/PIR, GCG/MSF, PHYLIP, GDE, or NEXUS.

Multiple Sequence Alignment

There are three main steps:

1. Do a pairwise alignment
2. Create a phylogenetic tree (or use a user-defined tree)
3. Use the phylogenetic tree to carry out a multiple alignment.

These are done automatically when you select "Do Complete Alignment". Other options are "Do Alignment from guide tree" and "Produce guide tree only".

Setting

Users can align the sequences using the default setting, but occasionally it may be useful to customize one's own parameters.

The main parameters are the gap opening penalty, and the gap extension penalty.

Multiple Sequence Alignment

A multiple sequence alignment (MSA) is a sequence alignment of three or more biological sequences, generally protein, DNA, or RNA. In many cases, the input set of query sequences are assumed to have an evolutionary relationship by which they share a lineage and are descended from a common ancestor.

From the resulting MSA, sequence homology can be inferred and phylogenetic analysis can be conducted to assess the sequences' shared evolutionary origins. Visual depictions of the alignment as in the image at right illustrate mutation events such as point mutations (single amino acid or nucleotide changes) that appear as differing characters in a single alignment column, and insertion or deletion mutations (indels or gaps) that appear as hyphens in one or more of the sequences in the alignment. Multiple sequence alignment is often used to assess sequence conservation of protein domains, tertiary and secondary structures, and even individual amino acids or nucleotides.

Multiple sequence alignment also refers to the process of aligning such a sequence set. Because three or more sequences of biologically relevant length can be difficult and are almost always time-consuming to align by hand, computational algorithms are used to produce and analyse the alignments. MSAs require more sophisticated methodologies than pairwise alignment because they are more computationally complex. Most multiple sequence alignment programs use heuristic methods rather than global optimization because identifying the optimal alignment between more than a few sequences of moderate length is prohibitively computationally expensive.

Dynamic Programming and Computational Complexity

A direct method for producing an MSA uses the dynamic programming technique to identify the globally optimal alignment solution. For proteins, this method usually involves two sets of parameters: a gap penalty and a substitution matrix assigning scores or probabilities to the alignment of each possible pair of amino acids based on the similarity of the amino acids' chemical properties and the evolutionary probability of the mutation.

For nucleotide sequences a similar gap penalty is used, but a much simpler substitution matrix, wherein only identical matches and mismatches are considered, is typical. The scores in the substitution matrix may be either all positive or a mix of positive and negative in the case of a global alignment, but must be both positive and negative, in the case of a local alignment.

For *n* individual sequences, the naive method requires constructing the *n*-dimensional equivalent of the matrix formed in standard pairwise sequence alignment. The search space thus increases exponentially with increasing *n* and is also strongly dependent on sequence length. Expressed with the big O notation commonly used to measure computational complexity, a naïve MSA takes *O(Length)* time to produce. To find the global optimum for *n* sequences this way has been shown to be an NP-complete problem.

In 1989, based on Carrillo-Lipman Algorithm, Altschul introduced a practical method that uses pairwise alignments to constrain the n-dimensional search space. In this approach pairwise dynamic programming alignments are performed on each pair of sequences in the query set, and only the space near the n-dimensional intersection of these alignments is searched for the n-way alignment. The MSA program optimizes the sum of all of the pairs of characters at each position in the alignment (the so-called *sum of pair* score) and has been implemented in a software program for constructing multiple sequence alignments.

Progressive Alignment Construction

The most widely used approach to multiple sequence alignments uses a heuristic search known as progressive technique (also known as the hierarchical or tree method), that builds up a final MSA by combining pairwise alignments beginning with the most similar pair and progressing to the most distantly related.

All progressive alignment methods require two stages: a first stage in which the relationships between the sequences are represented as a tree, called a *guide tree*, and a second step in which the MSA is built by adding the sequences sequentially to the growing MSA according to the guide tree. The initial *guide tree* is determined by an efficient clustering method such as neighbour-joining or UPGMA, and may use distances based on the number of identical two letter sub-sequences (as in FASTA rather than a dynamic programming alignment).

Progressive alignments cannot be globally optimal. The primary problem is that when errors are made at any stage in growing the MSA, these errors are then propagated through to the final result.

Performance is also particularly bad when all of the sequences in the set are rather distantly related. Most modern progressive methods modify their scoring function with a secondary weighting function that assigns scaling factors to individual members of the query set in a nonlinear fashion based on their phylogenetic distance from their nearest neighbours. This corrects for non-random selection of the sequences given to the alignment program. Progressive alignment methods are efficient enough to implement on a large scale for many (100s to 1000s) sequences. Progressive alignment services are commonly available on publicly accessible web servers so users need not locally install the applications of interest.

The most popular progressive alignment method has been the Clustal family, especially the weighted variant ClustalW to which access is provided by a large number of web portals including GenomeNet, EBI, and EMBNet. Different portals or implementations can vary in user interface and make different parameters accessible to the user. ClustalW is used extensively for phylogenetic tree construction, in spite of the author's explicit warnings that unedited alignments should not be used in such studies and as input for protein structure prediction by homology modelling. Another common progressive alignment method called T-Coffee is slower than Clustal and its derivatives but generally produces more accurate alignments for distantly related sequence sets.

T-Coffee calculates pairwise alignments by combining the direct alignment of the pair with indirect alignments that aligns each sequence of the pair to a third sequence. It uses the output from Clustal as well as another local alignment program LALIGN, which finds multiple regions of local alignment between two sequences. The resulting alignment and phylogenetic tree are used as a guide to produce new and more accurate weighting factors. Because progressive methods are heuristics that are not guaranteed to converge to a global optimum, alignment quality can be difficult to evaluate and their true biological significance can be obscure. A 2006, semi-progressive method that improves alignment quality and does not use a lossy heuristic while still running in polynomial time has been implemented in the program PSAlign.

Iterative Methods

A set of methods to produce MSAs while reducing the errors inherent in progressive methods are classified as "iterative" because they work similarly to progressive methods but repeatedly realign the initial sequences as well as adding new sequences to the growing MSA. One reason progressive methods are so strongly dependent on a high-quality initial alignment is the fact that these alignments are always incorporated into the final result-that is, once a sequence has been aligned into the MSA, its alignment is not considered further. This approximation improves efficiency at the cost of accuracy. By contrast, iterative methods can return to previously calculated pairwise alignments or sub-MSAs incorporating subsets of the query sequence as a means of optimizing a general objective function such as finding a high-quality alignment score.

A variety of subtly different iteration methods have been implemented and made available in software packages; reviews and comparisons have been useful but generally refrain from choosing a "best" technique. The software package PRRN/PRRP uses a hill-climbing algorithm to optimize its MSA alignment score and iteratively corrects both alignment weights and locally divergent or "gappy" regions of the growing MSA. PRRP performs best when refining an alignment previously constructed by a faster method.

Another iterative program, DIALIGN, takes an unusual approach of focusing narrowly on local alignments between sub-segments or sequence motifs without introducing a gap penalty. The alignment of individual motifs is then achieved with a matrix representation similar to a dot-matrix plot in a pairwise alignment. An alternative method that uses fast local alignments as anchor points or "seeds" for a slower global-alignment procedure is implemented in the CHAOS/DIALIGN suite.

A third popular iteration-based method called MUSCLE (multiple sequence alignment by log-expectation) improves on progressive methods with a more accurate distance measure to assess the relatedness of two sequences. The distance measure is updated between iteration stages (although, in its original form, MUSCLE contained only 2-3 iterations depending on whether refinement was enabled).

Hidden Markov models

Hidden Markov models are probabilistic models that can assign likelihoods to all possible combinations of gaps, matches, and mismatches to determine the most likely MSA or set of possible MSAs. HMMs can produce a single highest-scoring output but can also generate a family of possible alignments that can then be evaluated for biological significance. HMMs can produce both global and local alignments. Although HMM-based methods have been developed relatively recently, they offer significant improvements in computational speed, especially for sequences that contain overlapping regions.

Typical HMM-based methods work by representing an MSA as a form of directed acyclic graph known as a partial-order graph, which consists of a series of nodes representing possible entries in the columns of an MSA. In this representation a column that is absolutely conserved (that is, that all the sequences in the MSA share a particular character at a particular position) is coded as a single node with as many outgoing connections as there are possible characters in the next column of the alignment. In the terms of a typical hidden Markov model, the observed states are the individual alignment columns and the "hidden" states represent the presumed ancestral sequence from which the sequences in the query set are hypothesized to have descended.

An efficient search variant of the dynamic programming method, known as the Viterbi algorithm, is generally used to successively align the growing MSA to the next sequence in the query set to produce a new MSA. This is distinct from progressive alignment methods because the alignment of prior sequences is updated at each new sequence addition. However, like progressive methods, this technique can be influenced by the order in which the sequences in the query set are integrated into the alignment, especially when the sequences are distantly related.

Several software programs are available in which variants of HMM-based methods have been implemented and which are noted for their scalability and efficiency, although properly using an HMM method is more complex than using more common progressive methods.

The simplest is POA (Partial-Order Alignment); a similar but more generalized method is implemented in the packages SAM (Sequence Alignment and Modelling System). and HMMER. SAM has been used as a source of alignments for protein structure prediction to participate in the CASP structure prediction experiment and to develop a database of predicted proteins in the yeast species *S. cerevisiae*. HHsearch is a software package for the detection of remotely related protein sequences based on the pairwise comparison of HMMs. A server running HHsearch (HHpred) was by far the fastest of the

10 best automatic structure prediction servers in the CASP7 and CASP8 structure prediction competitions.

Genetic Algorithms and Simulated Annealing

Standard optimization techniques in computer science-both of which were inspired by, but do not directly reproduce, physical processes-have also been used in an attempt to more efficiently produce quality MSAs. One such technique, genetic algorithms, has been used for MSA production in an attempt to broadly simulate the hypothesized evolutionary process that gave rise to the divergence in the query set. The method works by breaking a series of possible MSAs into fragments and repeatedly rearranging those fragments with the introduction of gaps at varying positions. A general objective function is optimized during the simulation, most generally the "sum of pairs" maximization function introduced in dynamic programming-based MSA methods. A technique for protein sequences has been implemented in the software program SAGA (Sequence Alignment by Genetic Algorithm) and its equivalent in RNA is called RAGA.

The technique of simulated annealing, by which an existing MSA produced by another method is refined by a series of rearrangements designed to find more optimal regions of alignment space than the one the input alignment already occupies. Like the genetic algorithm method, simulated annealing maximizes an objective function like the sum-of-pairs function. Simulated annealing uses a metaphorical "temperature factor" that determines the rate at which rearrangements proceed and the likelihood of each rearrangement; typical usage alternates periods of high rearrangement rates with relatively low likelihood (to explore more distant regions of alignment space) with periods of lower rates and higher likelihoods to more thoroughly explore local minima near the newly "colonized" regions. This approach has been implemented in the program MSASA (Multiple Sequence Alignment by Simulated Annealing).

Motif Finding

Motif finding, also known as profile analysis, is a method of locating sequence motifs in global MSAs that is both a means of producing a better MSA and a means of producing a scoring matrix for use in searching other sequences for similar motifs. A variety of methods for isolating the motifs have been developed, but all are based on identifying short highly conserved patterns within the larger alignment and constructing a matrix similar to a substitution matrix that reflects the amino acid or nucleotide composition of each position in the putative motif. The alignment can then be refined using these matrices. In standard profile analysis, the matrix includes entries for each possible character as well as entries for gaps. Alternatively, statistical pattern-finding algorithms can identify motifs as a precursor to an MSA rather than as a derivation. In many cases when the query set contains only a small number of sequences or contains only highly related sequences, pseudocounts are added to normalize the distribution reflected in the scoring matrix. In particular, this corrects zero-probability entries in the matrix to values that are small but nonzero.

Blocks analysis is a method of motif finding that restricts motifs to ungapped regions in the alignment. Blocks can be generated from an MSA or they can be extracted from unaligned sequences using a precalculated set of common motifs previously generated from known gene families. Block scoring generally relies on the spacing of high-frequency characters rather than on the calculation of an explicit substitution matrix. The BLOCKS server provides an interactive method to locate such motifs in unaligned sequences.

Statistical pattern-matching has been implemented using both the expectation-maximization algorithm and the Gibbs sampler. One of the most common motif-finding tools, known as MEME, uses expectation maximization and hidden Markov methods to generate motifs that are then used as search tools by its companion MAST in the combined suite MEME/MAST.

Visualization and Editing Tools

The necessary use of heuristics for multiple alignment means that for an arbitrary set of proteins, there is always a good chance that an alignment will contain errors. These can arise because of unique insertions into one or more regions of sequences, or through some more complex evolutionary process leading to proteins that do not align easily by sequence alone. Multiple sequence alignment viewers enable alignments to be visually verified, often by inspecting the quality of alignment for annotated functional sites on two or more sequences. Many also enable the alignment to be edited to correct these (usually minor) errors, in order to obtain an optimal 'curated' alignment suitable for use in phylogenetic analysis or comparative modelling.

Use in Phylogenetics

Multiple sequence alignments can be used to create a phylogenetic tree. This is made possible by two reasons. The first is because functional domains that are known in annotated sequences can be used for alignment in non-annotated sequences. The other is that conserved regions known to be functionally important can be found. This makes it possible for multiple sequence alignments to be used to analyse and find evolutionary relationships through homology between sequences. Point mutations and insertion or deletion events (called indels) can be detected.

Multiple sequence alignments can also be used to identify functionally important sites, such as binding sites, active sites, or sites corresponding to other key functions, by locating conserved domains. When looking at multiple sequence alignments, it is useful to consider different aspects of the sequences when comparing sequences. These aspects include identity, similarity, and homology. Identity means that the sequences have identical residues at their respective positions.

On the other hand, similarity has to do with the sequences being compared having similar residues quantitatively. For example, in terms of nucleotide sequences, pyrimidines are considered similar to each other, as are purines. Similarity ultimately leads to homology, in that the more similar sequences are, the closer they are to being homologous. This homology in sequences, can then go on to help find common ancestry.

Sequence Alignment Software

This list of sequence alignment software is a compilation of software tools and web portals used in pairwise sequence alignment and multiple sequence alignment.

List of Alignment Visualization Software

Multiple alignment visualization tools typically serve four purposes:

- General comprehension of large-scale DNA or protein alignments
- Visualization of alignments for figures and publication.
- Manual editing and curation of automatically generated alignments.
- In depth analysis.

The rest of this article is focused on just multiple global alignments of homologous proteins. The first two are a natural consequence of the fact that most computational representations of alignments and their annotation are not human readable and best portrayed in the familiar sequence row and alignment column format, of which examples are widespread in the literature.

The third is a necessity because both Multiple sequence alignment and Structural alignment algorithms utilise heuristics which do not always perform perfectly. The fourth is a great example of how interactive graphical tools enable a worker involved in sequence analysis to conveniently execute a variety if different computational tools in order to explore an alignment's phylogenetic implications; or, to predict the structure and functional properties of a specific sequence (e.g. comparative modelling).

T-Coffee

T-Coffee (Tree-based Consistency Objective Function For alignment Evaluation) is a multiple sequence alignment software using a progressive approach. It generates a library of pairwise alignments to guide the multiple sequence alignment. It can also combine multiple sequences alignments obtained previously and in the latest versions can use structural information from PDB files (3D-Coffee). It has advanced features to evaluate the quality of the alignments and some capacity for identifying occurrence of motifs (Mocca). It produces alignment in the aln format (Clustal) by default, but can also produce PIR, MSF and FASTA format. The most common input formats are supported (FASTA, PIR).

Comparisons with other Alignment Software

While the default output is a Clustal-like format, it is sufficiently different from the output of ClustalW/X that many programs supporting Clustal format cannot read it; fortunately ClustalX *can* import T-Coffee output so the simplest fix for this issue is usually to import T-Coffee's output into ClustalX and then re-export. Another possibility is to request the strict Clustalw output format with the option "-output=clustalw_aln"

An important specificity of T-Coffee is its ability to combine different methods and different data types. In its latest version, T-Coffee can be used to combine protein sequences and structures, RNA sequences and structures. It can also run and combine the output of the most common sequence and structure alignment packages. T-Coffee comes along with a sophisticated sequence reformatting utility named seq_reformat.

Variations

M-Coffee

M-Coffee is a special mode of T-Coffee that makes it possible to combine the output of the most common multiple sequence alignment packages (Muscle, ClustalW, Mafft, ProbCons, etc). The resulting alignments are slightly better than the individual one, but most important the program indicates the alignment regions where the various packages agree upon. Regions of high agreement are usually well aligned.

Expresso and 3D-Coffee

These are special modes of T-Coffee making it possible to combine sequence and structures in an alignment. The structure based alignments can be carried out using the most common structural aligners such as TMalign, Mustang, and sap.

R-Coffee

R-Coffee is a special mode of T-Coffee making it possible to align RNA sequences while using secondary structure information.

Align-m

Align-m is a multiple sequence alignment program written by Ivo Van Walle.

Align-m has the ability to accomplish the following tasks:
- Multiple sequence alignment
- Include extra information to guide the sequence alignment
- Multiple structural alignment
- Homology modelling by (iteratively) combining sequence and structure alignment data
- 'Filtering' of BLAST or other pairwise alignments
- Combining many alignments into one consensus sequence
- Multiple genome alignment (can cope with rearrangements).

Dialign-TX

Dialign-TX is a multiple sequence alignment program written by Amarendran R. Subramanian and is substantial improvement of

Dialign-T by combining greedy and progressive alignment strategies in a new algorithm.

The original Dialign-T is a reimplementation of the multiple-alignment program Dialign. Due to several algorithmic improvements, it produces significantly better alignments on locally and globally related sequence sets than previous versions of Dialign. However, like the original implementation of the program, Dialign-T uses a straight-forward greedy approach to assemble multiple alignments from local pairwise sequence similarities. Such greedy approaches may be vulnerable to spurious random similarities and can therefore lead to suboptimal results. Dialign-TX is a substantial improvement of Dialign-T that combines the previous greedy algorithm with a progressive alignment approach.

Muscle

Muscle (multiple sequence comparison by log-expectation) is public domain, multiple sequence alignment software for protein and nucleotide sequences.

Muscle is often used as a replacement for Clustal, since it typically (but not always) gives better sequence alignments; in addition, Muscle is significantly faster than Clustal, especially for larger alignments (Edgar 2004).

Muscle is integrated into UGENE bioinformatics tool as a plugin.

ProbCons

ProbCons is an open source probabilistic consistency-based multiple alignment of amino acid sequences. It is an efficient protein multiple sequence alignment program, which has demonstrated a statistically significant improvement in accuracy compared to several leading alignment tools.

Ras Mol

RasMol is a computer program written for molecular graphics visualization intended and used primarily for the depiction and exploration of biological macromolecule structures, such as those found in the Protein Data Bank. It was originally developed by Roger Sayle in the early 90s.

Historically, it was an important tool for molecular biologists since the extremely optimized program allowed the software to run on (then) modestly powerful personal computers. Before RasMol, visualization software ran on graphics workstations that, due to their expense, were less accessible to scholars. RasMol has become an important educational tool as well as continuing to be an important tool for research in structural biology.

RasMol has a complex version history. Starting with the series of 2.7 versions, RasMol is licensed under a dual license (GPL or custom license *RASLIC*).

RasMol includes a language (for selecting certain protein chains, or changing colours etc). Jmol and Sirius has incorporated the RasMol scripting language into its commands.

Protein Databank (PDB) files can be downloaded for visualization from the Research Collaboratory for Structural Bioinformatics (RCSB) bank. These have been uploaded by researchers who have characterized the structure of molecules usually by X-ray crystallography or NMR spectroscopy.

Inter-process Communication

On UNIX platforms Rasmol can communicate with other programs via Tcl/Tk. Under Microsoft Windows, Dynamic Data Exchange (DDE) is used.

- multiple alignment program. The responsible Java class can be freely used in other applications.

Molscript

Molscript is probably the most widely used package for producing figures for publication derived from a PDB file normally as a postscript file on a white background. It was written by Per Kraulis at the University of Uppsala as part of his Ph.D. with Prof Alwyn Jones (of O fame). It was designed to produce figures in the style originally used by Jane Richardson with a helices as helical ribbons and b sheets as ribbon like arrows.

(Note: Molscript originally and primarily produces postscript files. The picture above is in JPEG format, which can be displayed directly by the browser. The default background in Molscript2 for this format is black and the line colour white so "background white;" and "set linecolour black;" have been added to the command file to get closer to the postscript appearance to look at the postscript file if your browser is configured to display it using an auxiliary program).

It was released in 1991 and the reference is:

Per J. Kraulis MOLSCRIPT: A Program to Produce Both Detailed and Schematic Plots of Protein Structures. Journal of Applied Crystallography (1991) 24, 946-950.

Due to it being a condition of the license that this reference is quoted in every paper using figures from Molscript it is already an Institute of Scientific Information citation classic (around 4000 references by Oct 1998). As can be seen from its level of use it is a very good piece of software and simple to use. It produces excellent printed figures, which even photocopy moderately well out of journals. However it does not produce the moodily lit and silkily rendered slides on a black background as well as say photographing the screen in O, or in a number of packages popular in the States. Lighting is a good way of presenting depth in a picture. *Raster3D* was developed by Merrit and Murphy to do this and was redesigned to take the output from Molscript as one possible implementation. There are programs in the raster3d package to assemble cartoons straight from PDB file and the output of other packages can be rendered using it but I will not be going into this in this session.

Ethan A. Merrit and Michael E.P. Murphy *Raster3D* Version 2.0 A Program for Photorealistic Molecular Graphics Acta Cryst. (1994) D50, 869-873.

D. Bacon and W.F.Anderson A fast algorithm for rendering space-filling molecule pictures. Journal of Molecular Graphics (1988) 6, 219-220. There are inevitably limitations to any software and a major limitation to Molscript was that electron density could not be drawn. Robert Esnouf (then at Oxford) adapted the code of Molscript to include map drawing routines (from a range of formats). He named this modified software *Bobscript*. He also included colour ramping that allows smooth changes of colouring of the molecule. This means that the molecule can be followed from beginning to end along a rainbow of colours. It also allows smooth colouring of the molecule by B factor, so that the most mobile bits can be say red and the least mobile bits blue. (Other properties can be substituted for B factor in the input file). Stereo plotting is carried out more explicitly.

The reference for Bobscript is:

R.M. Esnouf An extensively modified version of MolScript that includes greatly enhanced coloring capabilities. Journal of Molecular Graphics (1997), 15, 132-134

Finally about a year ago Per Kraulis released *Molscript V2*. This adds a large range of output formats including interactive OpenGL (allows rotation and determination of orientation also JPEG, EPS and PNG format outputs) and VRML (Virtual Reality Markup Language). He also implemented his own version of colour ramping. There is also the facility to handle 'external objects' which can be set up to be electron density.

This does not appear to match the ease of map plotting in Bobscript. Local implementation. All of the programs should run without the need for any further setting up on any of the Unix machines. (There is no need to invoke a *use* command). The current installed version will be displayed on starting the program. This may not always be the absolutely latest version if you visit the home pages for the software. To run molscript to produce a postscript file

molscript -ps < input.file > output.ps

To run molscript to produce an open gl file

molscript -gl <input.file

To run molscript and feed the result to Raster3d to produce a Silicon Graphics rgb file.

molscript -raster3d <input.file | render -sgi output.rgb

To run bobscript

bobscript <input.file>output.ps

Drawing Good Pictures

It is fairly easy to produce pictures quickly using molscript, but to convey what you want is much harder. This comes with practice and experience. The best way to learn is to look at other people's pictures. Think about what they show and don't show and whether it conveys what they say it does in the text. Try producing similar diagrams yourself.

Multiple Pictures and Stereo

Postscript output from Molscript and Bobscript can be positioned and sized on the page using the "area" command. Each command file can produce more than one picture. This is particularly useful for producing stereo pairs. In Bobscript there are explicit "leftstereo" and "rightstereo" commands; in Molscript small (+/- 3.0 degrees) rotations about y need to be added to the orientation commands.

Alternative Starting Files

Per Kraulis has released a program *Molauto*, which produces a starting molscript file from your pdb file. There are more options than with rasmol. These are all entered on the command line e.g.

Molauto -cpk xyz.pdb > xyz.inp

Means that any ligands are produced as CPK. Indeed the ability to handle ligands makes molauto better than rasmol. However it does not give you the view. To get that you must run molscript interactively

Molscript -gl <xyz.inp

And use the left mouse to print the orientation to your terminal window. This is entered using the "transform rotation" *3x3 matrix"* command.

Raster 3d Header

Raster3d used to be controlled by a file called "header.r3d" which had to be manually edited to control background and lighting. This is still required for Bobscript, but Molscript2 controls all these from the command file.

Alscript

Alscript is a program to format multiple sequence alignments in PostScript for publication and to assist in analysis. Alscript does not support point-and-click, but has a scripting language to allow complex effects.

Brief Description of Alscript

Alscript takes a multiple sequence alignment in AMPS (Barton &Sternberg, 1987, Barton, 1990) block-file format and a set of formatting commands and produces a PostScript file that may be printed on a PostScript laser printer, or viewed using a PostScript previewer (e.g. Sun Microsystem's PageView program). Clustal and GCG format multiple alignment files may also be used. Alscript is NOT a multiple sequence alignment program, nor is it an alignment editor.

Given a block-file and pointsize (character width/height), Alscript calculates how many residues can be fitted across the page, and how many sequences will fit down the page, it then prints the alignment at the chosen pointsize on as many pages as are needed.

Running ALSCRIPT with a smaller or larger pointsize will automatically re-scale the alignment to fit on fewer or more pages as appropriate. The actual page dimensions may be re-set to any value, so if you have access to an A3 PostScript printer, or typesetting machine, alignments can readily be scaled to maximise the available space. Each output page has three basic regions.

The left hand edge contains identifier codes for each sequence. The main part of the page holds the alignment, and the top part, the position numbers and tick marks. Alscript commands make use of a character coordinate system for font changes, and other formatting commands. Thus, any residue in the alignment may be referred to by its sequence position number (x-axis) and sequence number (y-axis), similarly, ranges of residue positions, or sequences may also be defined in the character coordinate system.

The basic Alscript commands allow the following functionality:

Fonts: Any PostScript font at any size may be defined and used on individual residues, regions or identifier codes.

Boxing: Simple rectangular boxes may be drawn around any part of the alignment. Particular residue types may be selected and automatically "surrounded" by lines. For example, if the characters 'G' and 'P' are selected, then lines will not be drawn between G and P characters, but only where G and P border with other characters.

Shading: Grey shading of any level from black to white may be applied to any region of the alignment, either as a rectangular region, or as residue specific shading. e.g. "shade all Cys residues between positions 6 and 30"

Text: Specific text strings may be added to the alignment at any position and in any font or font size.

Lines: Horizontal or vertical lines may be drawn to the left, right, top or bottom of any residue position or group of positions.

Colour: Characters or character backgrounds may be independently coloured.

The example block file "example1.blc" and command file "example1.als" illustrate most of these commands in action.

Although written with the aim of producing figures for journal submission, ALSCRIPT may be used as a tool for interpreting multiple sequence alignments. For example, the boxing, shading and font changing facilities can be applied to highlight amino acids of a particular type and thus draw attention to clusters of positive or negative charge, hydrophobics, etc.

Phylip

Phylip (Phylogeny Inference Package) is a free computational phylogenetics package of programs for inferring evolutionary trees (phylogenies). The name is an acronym for *PHYLogeny Inference Package*. It consists of 35 portable programs, i.e. the source code is written in C and precompiled executables are available for Windows (95/98/NT/2000/me/XP), Mac OS 8 and 9, Mac OS X, and Linux systems. Complete documentation is written for all the programs in the package and is part of the package.

The author of this package is Joseph Felsenstein, Professor in the Department of Genome Sciences and the Department of Biology at the University of Washington, Seattle.

Methods (implemented by each program) that are available in the package include parsimony, distance matrix, and likelihood methods, including bootstrapping and consensus trees. Data types that can be handled include molecular sequences, gene frequencies, restriction sites and fragments, distance matrices, and discrete characters.

Each program is controlled through a menu, which asks the users which options they want to set, and allows them to start the computation. The data is read into the program from a text file, which the user can prepare using any word processor or text editor (but it is important that this text file not be in the special format of that word processor — it should instead be in *flat ASCII* or *Text Only* format).

Some sequence analysis programs such as the ClustalW alignment program can write data files in the Phylip format. Most of the programs look for the data in a file called *infile* — if they do not find this file they then ask the user to type in the file name of the data file.

Output is written onto files with names like outfile and outtree. Trees written onto outtree are in the Newick format, an informal standard agreed to in 1986 by authors of a number of major phylogeny packages.

Phylip Programs

The programs listed in PHYLIP are:

Program Name	Description
protpars	Estimates phylogenies of protein sequences using the Parsimony Method
dnapars	Estimates phylogenies of DNA sequences using the parsimony method.
dnapenny	DNA parsimony branch and bound method. Finds all of the most parsimonious phylogenies for nucleic acid sequences by branch-and-bound search
dnamove	Interactive construction of phylogenies from nucleic acid sequences, with their evaluation by DNA parsimony method, with compatibility and display of reconstructed ancestral bases.
dnacomp	Estimates phylogenies from nucleic acid sequence data using the compatibility criterion.
dnaml	Estimates phylogenies from nucleotide sequences using the maximum likelihood method.
dnamlk	DNA maximum likelihood method with molecular clock. Using both dnaml and dnamlk together permits a likelihood-ratio test for the molecular clock hypothesis.
proml	Estimates phylogenies from protein amino acid sequences by using the maximum likelihood method.
promlk	Protein sequence maximum likelihood method with molecular clock.
restml	Estimation of phylogenies by maximum likelihood using restriction sites data (not from restriction fragments but from the presence or absence of individual sites).
dnainvar	For nucleic acid sequence data on four species, computes Lake's and Cavender's phylogenetic invariants, which test alternative tree topologies.
dnadist	DNA distance method which computes four different distances between species from nucleic acid sequences. The distances can then be used in the distance matrix programs.
protdist	Protein sequence distance method which computes a distance measure for protein sequences, using maximum likelihood estimates based on the Dayhoff PAM matrix, Kimura's 1983 approximation to it, or a model based on the genetic code plus a constraint on changing to a different category of amino acid.

Contd...

Program Name	Description
restdist	Distances calculated from restriction sites data or restriction fragments data.
seqboot	Bootstrapping/Jackknifing program. Reads in a data set, and produces multiple data sets from it by bootstrap resampling.
fitch	Fitch-Margoliash distance matrix method. Estimates phylogenies from distance matrix data under the "additive tree model" according to which the distances are expected to equal the sums of branch lengths between the species.
kitsch	Fitch-Margoliash distance matrix method with molecular clock. Estimates phylogenies from distance matrix data under the "ultrametric" model which is the same as the additive tree model except that an evolutionary clock is assumed.
neighbour	An implementation of the Neighbour-Joining method and the UPGMA method.
contml	Maximum likelihood continuous characters and gene frequencies. Estimates phylogenies from gene frequency data by maximum likelihood under a model in which all divergence is due to genetic drift in the absence of new mutations. This program can also do maximum likelihood analysis of continuous characters that evolve by a Brownian Motion model, assuming that the characters evolve at equal rates and in an uncorrelated fashion. Does not take into account the correlations of characters.
contrast	Reads a tree from a tree file, and a data set with continuous characters data, and produces the independent contrasts for those characters, for use in any multivariate statistics package.
gendist	Genetic distance program which computes one of three different genetic distance formulas from gene frequency data
pars	Unordered multistate discrete-characters parsimony method.
mix	Estimates phylogenies by some parsimony methods for discrete character data with two states (0 and 1). Allows use of the Wagner parsimony method, the Camin-Sokal parsimony method, or arbitrary mixtures of these.

Contd...

Program Name	Description
penny	Branch and bound mixed method which finds all of the most parsimonious phylogenies for discrete-character data with two states, for the Wagner, Camin-Sokal, and mixed parsimony criteria using the branch-and-bound method of exact search.
move	Interactive construction of phylogenies from discrete character data with two states (0 and 1). Evaluates parsimony and compatibility criteria for those phylogenies and displays reconstructed states throughout the tree.
dollop	Estimates phylogenies by the Dollo or polymorphism parsimony criteria for discrete character data with two states (0 and 1).
dolpenny	Finds all most parsimonious phylogenies for discrete-character data with two states, for the Dollo or polymorphism parsimony criteria using the branch-and-bound method of exact search.
dolmove	Interactive construction of phylogenies from discrete character data with two states (0 and 1) using the Dollo or polymorphism parsimony criteria. Evaluates parsimony and compatibility criteria for those phylogenies and displays reconstructed states throughout the tree.
clique	Finds the largest clique of mutually compatible characters, and the phylogeny which they recommend, for discrete character data with two states (0 and 1). The largest clique (or all cliques within a given size range of the largest one) are found by a very fast branch and bound search method.
factor	Character recoding program which takes discrete multistate data with character state trees and produces the corresponding data set with two states (0 and 1).
drawgram	Rooted tree drawing program which plots rooted phylogenies, cladograms, and phenograms in a wide variety of user-controllable formats. The program is interactive and allows previewing of the tree on PC or Macintosh graphics screens, and Tektronix or Digital graphics terminals.
drawtree	Unrooted tree drawing program similar to DRAWGRAM, but plots unrooted phylogenies..

Contd...

Program Name	Description
consense	Consensus tree program which Computes consensus trees by the majority-rule consensus tree method, which also allows one to easily find the strict consensus tree. Is not able to compute the Adams consensus tree
treedist	Computes the Robinson-Foulds symmetric difference distance between trees, which allows for differences in tree topology.
retree	interactive tree rearrangement program which reads in a tree (with branch lengths if necessary) and allows you to reroot the tree, to flip branches, to change species names and branch lengths, and then write the result out. Can be used to convert between rooted and unrooted trees.

Chapter 5

Bioinformatics Sequence Alignments

In bioinformatics, a sequence alignment is a way of arranging the sequences of DNA, RNA, or protein to identify regions of similarity that may be a consequence of functional, structural, or evolutionary relationships between the sequences. Aligned sequences of nucleotide or amino acid residues are typically represented as rows within a matrix. Gaps are inserted between the residues so that identical or similar characters are aligned in successive columns. A sequence alignment, produced by ClustalW, of two human zinc finger proteins, identified on the left by GenBank accession number.

Interpretation

If two sequences in an alignment share a common ancestor, mismatches can be interpreted as point mutations and gaps as indels (that is, insertion or deletion mutations) introduced in one or both lineages in the time since they diverged from one another. In sequence alignments of proteins, the degree of similarity between amino acids occupying a particular position in the sequence can be interpreted as a rough measure of how conserved a particular region or sequence motif is among lineages. The absence of substitutions, or the presence of only very conservative substitutions (that is, the substitution of amino acids whose side chains have similar biochemical properties) in a particular region of the sequence, suggest that this region has structural or functional importance. Although DNA and RNA nucleotide bases are more similar to each other than are amino acids, the conservation of base pairs can indicate a similar functional or structural role.

Alignment Methods

Very short or very similar sequences can be aligned by hand. However, most interesting problems require the alignment of lengthy, highly variable or extremely numerous sequences that cannot be aligned solely by human effort. Instead, human knowledge is applied in constructing algorithms to produce high-quality sequence alignments, and occasionally in adjusting the final results to reflect patterns that are difficult to represent algorithmically (especially in the case of nucleotide sequences).

Computational approaches to sequence alignment generally fall into two categories: *global alignments* and *local alignments*. Calculating a global alignment is a form of global optimization that "forces" the alignment to span the entire length of all query sequences. By contrast, local alignments identify regions of similarity within long sequences that are often widely divergent overall. Local alignments are often preferable, but can be more difficult to calculate because of the additional challenge of identifying the regions of similarity. A variety of computational algorithms have been applied to the sequence alignment problem, including slow but formally optimizing methods like dynamic programming, and efficient, but not as thorough heuristic algorithms or probabilistic methods designed for large-scale database search.

Representations

Alignments are commonly represented both graphically and in text format. In almost all sequence alignment representations, sequences are written in rows arranged so that aligned residues appear in successive columns. In text formats, aligned columns containing identical or similar characters are indicated with a system of conservation symbols. As in the image above, an asterisk or pipe symbol is used to show identity between two columns; other less common symbols include a colon for conservative substitutions and a period for semiconservative substitutions.

Many sequence visualization programs also use colour to display information about the properties of the individual sequence elements; in DNA and RNA sequences, this equates to assigning each nucleotide its own colour. In protein alignments, such as the one in the image above, colour is often used to indicate amino acid properties to aid in judging the conservation of a given amino acid substitution. For multiple sequences the last row in each column is often the consensus sequence determined by the alignment; the consensus sequence is also often represented in graphical format with a sequence logo in which the size of each nucleotide or amino acid letter corresponds to its degree of conservation.

Sequence alignments can be stored in a wide variety of text-based file formats, many of which were originally developed in conjunction with a specific alignment program or implementation. Most web-based tools allow a limited number of input and output formats, such as FASTA format and GenBank format and the output is not easily editable. Several conversion programs are available, READSEQ or EMBOSS having a graphical interfaces or command line interfaces, while several programming packages like BioPerl, BioRuby provide functions to do this.

Global and Local Alignments

Global alignments, which attempt to align every residue in every sequence, are most useful when the sequences in the query set are similar and of roughly equal size. (This does not mean global alignments cannot end in gaps.) A general global alignment technique is the Needleman-Wunsch algorithm, which is based on dynamic programming. Local alignments are more useful for dissimilar sequences that are suspected to contain regions of similarity or similar sequence motifs within their larger sequence context. The Smith-Waterman algorithm is a general local alignment method also based on dynamic programming. With sufficiently similar sequences, there is no difference between local and global alignments.

Hybrid methods, known as semiglobal or "glocal" methods, attempt to find the best possible alignment that includes the start and end of one or the other sequence. This can be especially useful when the downstream part of one sequence overlaps with the upstream part of the other sequence. In this case, neither global nor local alignment is entirely appropriate: a global alignment would attempt to force the alignment to extend beyond the region of overlap, while a local alignment might not fully cover the region of overlap.

Pairwise Alignment

Pairwise sequence alignment methods are used to find the best-matching piecewise (local) or global alignments of two query sequences. Pairwise alignments can only be used between two sequences at a time, but they are efficient to calculate and are often used for methods that do not require extreme precision (such as searching a database for sequences with high similarity to a query). The three primary methods of producing pairwise alignments are dot-matrix methods, dynamic programming, and word methods; however, multiple sequence alignment techniques can also align pairs of sequences.

Although each method has its individual strengths and weaknesses, all three pairwise methods have difficulty with highly repetitive sequences of low information content- especially where the number of repetitions differ in the two sequences to be aligned. One way of quantifying the utility of a given pairwise alignment is the 'maximum unique match', or the longest subsequence that occurs in both query sequence. Longer MUM sequences typically reflect closer relatedness.

Dot-matrix Methods

The dot-matrix approach, which implicitly produces a family of alignments for individual sequence regions, is qualitative and conceptually simple, though time-consuming to analyse on a large scale. In the absence of noise, it can be easy to visually identify certain sequence features—such as insertions, deletions, repeats, or inverted repeats—from a dot-matrix plot.

To construct a dot-matrix plot, the two sequences are written along the top row and leftmost column of a two-dimensional matrix and a dot is placed at any point where the characters in the appropriate columns match—this is a typical recurrence plot. Some implementations vary the size or intensity of the dot depending on the degree of similarity of the two characters, to accommodate conservative substitutions. The dot plots of very closely related sequences will appear as a single line along the matrix's main diagonal.

Problems with dot plots as an information display technique include: noise, lack of clarity, non-intuitiveness, difficulty extracting match summary statistics and match positions on the two sequences. There is also much wasted space where the match data is inherently duplicated across the diagonal and most of the actual area of the plot is taken up by either empty space or noise, and, finally, dot-plots are limited to two sequences. None of these limitations apply to Miropeats alignment diagrams but they have their own particular flaws.

Dot plots can also be used to assess repetitiveness in a single sequence. A sequence can be plotted against itself and regions that share significant similarities will appear as lines off the main diagonal.

This effect can occur when a protein consists of multiple similar structural domains.

Dynamic Programming

The technique of dynamic programming can be applied to produce global alignments via the Needleman-Wunsch algorithm, and local alignments via the Smith-Waterman algorithm. In typical usage, protein alignments use a substitution matrix to assign scores to amino-acid matches or mismatches, and a gap penalty for matching an amino acid in one sequence to a gap in the other.

DNA and RNA alignments may use a scoring matrix, but in practice often simply assign a positive match score, a negative mismatch score, and a negative gap penalty. (In standard dynamic programming, the score of each amino acid position is independent of the identity of its neighbours, and therefore base stacking effects are not taken into account. However, it is possible to account for such effects by modifying the algorithm.)

A common extension to standard linear gap costs, is the usage of two different gap penalties for opening a gap and for extending a gap. Typically the former is much larger than the latter, e.g. -10 for gap open and -2 for gap extension. Thus, the number of gaps in an alignment is usually reduced and residues and gaps are kept together, which typically makes more biological sense. The Gotoh algorithm implements affine gap costs by using three matrices.

Dynamic programming can be useful in aligning nucleotide to protein sequences, a task complicated by the need to take into account frameshift mutations (usually insertions or deletions). The framesearch method produces a series of global or local pairwise alignments between a query nucleotide sequence and a search set of protein sequences, or vice versa. Its ability to evaluate frameshifts offset by an arbitrary number of nucleotides makes the method useful for sequences containing large numbers of indels, which can be very difficult to align with more efficient heuristic methods.

In practice, the method requires large amounts of computing power or a system whose architecture is specialized for dynamic programming. The BLAST and EMBOSS suites provide basic tools for creating translated alignments (though some of these approaches take advantage of side-effects of sequence searching capabilities of the tools). More general methods are available from both commercial sources, such as *FrameSearch*, distributed as part of the Accelrys GCG package, and Open Source software such as Genewise.

The dynamic programming method is guaranteed to find an optimal alignment given a particular scoring function; however, identifying a good scoring function is often an empirical rather than a theoretical matter. Although dynamic programming is extensible to more than two sequences, it is prohibitively slow for large numbers of or extremely long sequences.

Word Methods

Word methods, also known as k-tuple methods, are heuristic methods that are not guaranteed to find an optimal alignment solution, but are significantly more efficient than dynamic programming. These methods are especially useful in large-scale database searches where it is understood that a large proportion of the candidate sequences will have essentially no significant match with the query sequence. Word methods are best known for their implementation in the database search tools FASTA and the BLAST family.

Word methods identify a series of short, nonoverlapping subsequences ("words") in the query sequence that are then matched to candidate database sequences. The relative positions of the word in the two sequences being compared are subtracted to obtain an offset; this will indicate a region of alignment if multiple distinct words produce the same offset. Only if this region is detected do these methods apply more sensitive alignment criteria; thus, many unnecessary comparisons with sequences of no appreciable similarity are eliminated.

In the FASTA method, the user defines a value k to use as the word length with which to search the database. The method is slower but more sensitive at lower values of k, which are also preferred for searches involving a very short query sequence. The BLAST family of search methods provides a number of algorithms optimized for particular types of queries, such as searching for distantly related sequence matches. BLAST was developed to provide a faster alternative to FASTA without sacrificing much accuracy; like FASTA, BLAST uses a word search of length k, but evaluates only the most significant word matches, rather than every word match as does FASTA. Most BLAST implementations use a fixed default word length that is optimized for the query and database type, and that is changed only under special circumstances, such as when searching with repetitive or very short query sequences. Implementations can be found via a number of web portals, such as EMBL FASTA and NCBI BLAST.

Multiple Sequence Alignment

Multiple sequence alignment is an extension of pairwise alignment to incorporate more than two sequences at a time. Multiple alignment methods try to align all of the sequences in a given query set. Multiple alignments are often used in identifying conserved sequence regions across a group of sequences hypothesized to be evolutionarily related. Such conserved sequence motifs can be used in conjunction with structural and mechanistic information to locate the catalytic active sites of enzymes.

Alignments are also used to aid in establishing evolutionary relationships by constructing phylogenetic trees. Multiple sequence alignments are computationally difficult to produce and most formulations of the problem lead to NP-complete combinatorial optimization problems. Nevertheless, the utility of these alignments in bioinformatics has led to the development of a variety of methods suitable for aligning three or more sequences.

Dynamic Programming

The technique of dynamic programming is theoretically applicable to any number of sequences; however, because it is computationally expensive in both time and memory, it is rarely used for more than three or four sequences in its most basic form. This method requires constructing the n-dimensional equivalent of the sequence matrix formed from two sequences, where n is the number of sequences in the query.

Standard dynamic programming is first used on all pairs of query sequences and then the "alignment space" is filled in by considering possible matches or gaps at intermediate positions, eventually constructing an alignment essentially between each two-sequence alignment. Although this technique is computationally expensive, its guarantee of a global optimum solution is useful in cases where only a few sequences need to be aligned accurately. One method for reducing the computational demands of dynamic programming, which relies on the "sum of pairs" objective function, has been implemented in the MSA software package.

Progressive Methods

Progressive, hierarchical, or tree methods generate a multiple sequence alignment by first aligning the most similar sequences and then adding successively less related sequences or groups to the alignment until the entire query set has been incorporated into the solution. The initial tree describing the sequence relatedness is based on pairwise comparisons that may include heuristic pairwise alignment methods similar to FASTA.

Progressive alignment results are dependent on the choice of "most related" sequences and thus can be sensitive to inaccuracies in the initial pairwise alignments. Most progressive multiple sequence alignment methods additionally weight the sequences in the query set according to their relatedness, which reduces the likelihood of making a poor choice of initial sequences and thus improves alignment accuracy.

Many variations of the Clustal progressive implementation are used for multiple sequence alignment, phylogenetic tree construction, and as input for protein structure prediction. A slower but more accurate variant of the progressive method is known as T-Coffee.

Iterative Methods

Iterative methods attempt to improve on the weak point of the progressive methods, the heavy dependence on the accuracy of the initial pairwise alignments. Iterative methods optimize an objective function based on a selected alignment scoring method by assigning an initial global alignment and then realigning sequence subsets. The realigned subsets are then themselves aligned to produce the next iteration's multiple sequence alignment. Various ways of selecting the sequence subgroups and objective function are reviewed in.

Motif Finding

Motif finding, also known as profile analysis, constructs global multiple sequence alignments that attempt to align short conserved sequence motifs among the sequences in the query set. This is usually done by first constructing a general global multiple sequence alignment, after which the highly conserved regions are isolated and used to construct a set of profile matrices. The profile matrix for each conserved region is arranged like a scoring matrix but its frequency counts for each amino acid or nucleotide at each position are derived from the conserved region's character distribution rather than from a more general empirical distribution. The profile matrices are then used to search other sequences for occurrences of the motif they characterize. In cases where the original data set contained a small number of sequences, or only highly related sequences, pseudocounts are added to normalize the character distributions represented in the motif.

Techniques Inspired by Computer Science

A variety of general optimization algorithms commonly used in computer science have also been applied to the multiple sequence alignment problem. Hidden Markov models have been used to produce probability scores for a family of possible multiple sequence alignments for a given query set; although early HMM-based methods produced underwhelming performance, later applications have found them especially effective in detecting remotely related sequences because they are less susceptible to noise created by conservative or semiconservative substitutions. Genetic algorithms and simulated annealing have also been used in optimizing multiple sequence alignment scores as judged by a scoring function like the sum-of-pairs method. More complete details and software packages can be found in the main article multiple sequence alignment.

Structural Alignment

Structural alignments, which are usually specific to protein and sometimes RNA sequences, use information about the secondary and tertiary structure of the protein or RNA molecule to aid in aligning the sequences. These methods can be used for two or more sequences and typically produce local alignments; however, because they depend on the availability of structural information, they can only be used for sequences whose corresponding structures are known (usually through X-ray crystallography or NMR spectroscopy). Because both protein and RNA structure is more evolutionarily conserved than sequence, structural alignments can be more reliable between sequences that are very distantly related and that have diverged so extensively that sequence comparison cannot reliably detect their similarity.

Structural alignments are used as the "gold standard" in evaluating alignments for homology-based protein structure prediction because they explicitly align regions of the protein sequence that are structurally similar rather than relying exclusively on sequence information.

However, clearly structural alignments cannot be used in structure prediction because at least one sequence in the query set is the target to be modelled, for which the structure is not known. It has been shown that, given the structural alignment between a target and a template sequence, highly accurate models of the target protein sequence can be produced; a major stumbling block in homology-based structure prediction is the production of structurally accurate alignments given only sequence information.

DALI

The DALI method, or distance matrix alignment, is a fragment-based method for constructing structural alignments based on contact similarity patterns between successive hexapeptides in the query sequences. It can generate pairwise or multiple alignments and identify a query sequence's structural neighbours in the Protein Data Bank (PDB). It has been used to construct the FSSP structural alignment database (Fold classification based on Structure-Structure alignment of Proteins, or Families of Structurally Similar Proteins). A DALI webserver can be accessed at EBI DALI and the FSSP is located at The Dali Database.

SSAP

SSAP (sequential structure alignment program) is a dynamic programming-based method of structural alignment that uses atom-to-atom vectors in structure space as comparison points. It has been extended since its original description to include multiple as well as pairwise alignments, and has been used in the construction of the CATH (Class, Architecture, Topology, Homology) hierarchical database classification of protein folds. The CATH database can be accessed at CATH Protein Structure Classification.

Combinatorial Extension

The combinatorial extension method of structural alignment generates a pairwise structural alignment by using local geometry to align short fragments of the two proteins being analysed and then assembles these fragments into a larger alignment. Based on measures such as rigid-body root mean square distance, residue distances, local secondary structure, and surrounding environmental features such as residue neighbour hydrophobicity, local alignments called "aligned fragment pairs" are generated and used to build a similarity matrix representing all possible structural alignments within predefined cutoff criteria. A path from one protein structure state to the other is then traced through the matrix by extending the growing alignment one fragment at a time.

The optimal such path defines the combinatorial-extension alignment. A web-based server implementing the method and providing a database of pairwise alignments of structures in the Protein Data Bank is located at the Combinatorial Extension website.

Phylogenetic Analysis

Phylogenetics and sequence alignment are closely related fields due to the shared necessity of evaluating sequence relatedness. The field of phylogenetics makes extensive use of sequence alignments in the construction and interpretation of phylogenetic trees, which are used to classify the evolutionary relationships between homologous genes represented in the genomes of divergent species. The degree to which sequences in a query set differ is qualitatively related to the sequences' evolutionary distance from one another.

Roughly speaking, high sequence identity suggests that the sequences in question have a comparatively young most recent common ancestor, while low identity suggests that the divergence is more ancient. This approximation, which reflects the "molecular clock" hypothesis that a roughly constant rate of evolutionary change can be used to extrapolate the elapsed time since two genes first diverged (that is, the coalescence time), assumes that the effects of mutation and selection are constant across sequence lineages.

Therefore it does not account for possible difference among organisms or species in the rates of DNA repair or the possible functional conservation of specific regions in a sequence. (In the case of nucleotide sequences, the molecular clock hypothesis in its most basic form also discounts the difference in acceptance rates between silent mutations that do not alter the meaning of a given codon and other mutations that result in a different amino acid being incorporated into the protein.) More statistically accurate methods allow the evolutionary rate on each branch of the phylogenetic tree to vary, thus producing better estimates of coalescence times for genes.

Progressive multiple alignment techniques produce a phylogenetic tree by necessity because they incorporate sequences into the growing alignment in order of relatedness. Other techniques that assemble multiple sequence alignments and phylogenetic trees score and sort trees first and calculate a multiple sequence alignment from the highest-scoring tree. Commonly used methods of phylogenetic tree construction are mainly heuristic because the problem of selecting the optimal tree, like the problem of selecting the optimal multiple sequence alignment, is NP-hard.

Assessment of Significance

Sequence alignments are useful in bioinformatics for identifying sequence similarity, producing phylogenetic trees, and developing homology models of protein structures. However, the biological relevance of sequence alignments is not always clear. Alignments are often assumed to reflect a degree of evolutionary change between sequences descended from a common ancestor; however, it is formally possible that convergent evolution can occur to produce apparent similarity between proteins that are evolutionarily unrelated but perform similar functions and have similar structures.

In database searches such as BLAST, statistical methods can determine the likelihood of a particular alignment between sequences or sequence regions arising by chance given the size and composition of the database being searched. These values can vary significantly depending on the search space. In particular, the likelihood of finding a given alignment by chance increases if the database consists only of sequences from the same organism as the query sequence. Repetitive sequences in the database or query can also distort both the search results and the assessment of statistical significance; BLAST automatically filters such repetitive sequences in the query to avoid apparent hits that are statistical artifacts.

Methods of statistical significance estimation for gapped sequence alignments are available in the literature.

Assessment of Credibility

Statistical significance indicates the probability that an alignment of a given quality could arise by chance, but does not indicate how much superior a given alignment is to alternative alignments of the same sequences. Measures of alignment credibility indicate the extent to which the best scoring alignments for a given pair of sequences are substantially similar. Methods of alignment credibility estimation for gapped sequence alignments are available in the literature.

Scoring Functions

The choice of a scoring function that reflects biological or statistical observations about known sequences is important to producing good alignments. Protein sequences are frequently aligned using substitution matrices that reflect the probabilities of given character-to-character substitutions. A series of matrices called PAM matrices (Point Accepted Mutation matrices, originally defined by Margaret Dayhoff and sometimes referred to as "Dayhoff matrices") explicitly encode evolutionary approximations regarding the rates and probabilities of particular amino acid mutations.

Another common series of scoring matrices, known as BLOSUM (Blocks Substitution Matrix), encodes empirically derived substitution probabilities. Variants of both types of matrices are used to detect sequences with differing levels of divergence, thus allowing users of BLAST or FASTA to restrict searches to more closely related matches or expand to detect more divergent sequences.

Gap penalties account for the introduction of a gap- on the evolutionary model, an insertion or deletion mutation- in both nucleotide and protein sequences, and therefore the penalty values should be proportional to the expected rate of such mutations. The quality of the alignments produced therefore depends on the quality of the scoring function.

It can be very useful and instructive to try the same alignment several times with different choices for scoring matrix and/or gap penalty values and compare the results. Regions where the solution is weak or non-unique can often be identified by observing which regions of the alignment are robust to variations in alignment parameters.

Other Biological Uses

Sequenced RNA, such as expressed sequence tags and full-length mRNAs, can be aligned to a sequenced genome to find where there are genes and get information about alternative splicing and RNA editing. Sequence alignment is also a part of genome assembly, where sequences are aligned to find overlap so that *contigs* (long stretches of sequence) can be formed. Another use is SNP analysis, where sequences from different individuals are aligned to find single basepairs that are often different in a population.

Non-biological Uses

The methods used for biological sequence alignment have also found applications in other fields, most notably in natural language processing and in social sciences. Techniques that generate the set of elements from which words will be selected in natural-language generation algorithms have borrowed multiple sequence alignment techniques from bioinformatics to produce linguistic versions of computer-generated mathematical proofs.

In the field of historical and comparative linguistics, sequence alignment has been used to partially automate the comparative method by which linguists traditionally reconstruct languages. Business and marketing research has also applied multiple sequence alignment techniques in analysing series of purchases over time.

Software

A more complete list of available software categorized by algorithm and alignment type is available at sequence alignment software, but common software tools used for general sequence alignment tasks include ClustalW and T-coffee for alignment, and BLAST and FASTA3x for database searching. Alignment algorithms and software can be directly compared to one another using a standardized set of benchmark reference multiple sequence alignments known as BAliBASE.

The data set consists of structural alignments, which can be considered a standard against which purely sequence-based methods are compared. The relative performance of many common alignment methods on frequently encountered alignment problems has been tabulated and selected results published online at BAliBASE. A comprehensive list of BAliBASE scores for many (currently 12) different alignment tools can be computed within the protein workbench STRAP.

Needleman-Wunsch

The Needleman–Wunsch algorithm performs a global alignment on two sequences (called A and B here). It is commonly used in bioinformatics to align protein or nucleotide sequences. The algorithm was published in 1970 by Saul B. Needleman and Christian D. Wunsch.

The Needleman–Wunsch algorithm is an example of dynamic programming, and was the first application of dynamic programming to biological sequence comparison.

Smith-waterman

The Smith-Waterman algorithm is a well-known algorithm for performing local sequence alignment; that is, for determining similar regions between two nucleotide or protein sequences. Instead of looking at the total sequence, the Smith-Waterman algorithm compares segments of all possible lengths and optimizes the similarity measure.

Background

The algorithm was first proposed by Temple F. Smith and Michael S. Waterman in 1981. Like the Needleman-Wunsch algorithm, of which it is a variation, Smith-Waterman is a dynamic programming algorithm. As such, it has the desirable property that it is guaranteed to find the optimal local alignment with respect to the scoring system being used (which includes the substitution matrix and the gap-scoring scheme).

The main difference to the Needleman-Wunsch algorithm is that negative scoring matrix cells are set to zero, which renders the (thus positively scoring) local alignments visible. Backtracking starts at the highest scoring matrix cell and proceeds until a cell with score zero is encountered, yielding the highest scoring local alignment. One does not actually implement the algorithm as described because improved alternatives are now available that have better scaling (Gotoh, 1982) and are more accurate.

Algorithm Explanation

A matrix H is built as follows:

$H(i,0) = 0,\ 0 \leq i \leq m$

$H(0,j) = 0,\ 0 \leq j \leq n$

if $a_i = b_j\ w\ (a_i,b_j) = w$ (match) or if $a_i! = b_j\ w\ (a_i,b_j) = w$ (mismatch);
Where:

- a,b = Strings over the Alphabet ε
- m = length(a)
- n = length(b)
- $H(i,j)$ - is the maximum Similarity-Score between a suffix of a[1...i] and a suffix of b[1...j]
- , '·' is the gap-scoring scheme.

Example

- Sequence 1 = ACACACTA
- Sequence 2 = AGCACACA
- w(match) = +2
- $w(a, -) = w(-,b) = w(mismatch) = -1$

To obtain the optimum local alignment, we start with the highest value in the matrix (i,j). Then, we go backwards to one of positions (i-1,j), (i,j-1), and (i-1,j-1) depending on the direction of movement used to construct the matrix. We keep the process until we reach a matrix cell with zero value, or the value in position (0,0).

In the example, the highest value corresponds to the cell in position (8,8). The walk back corresponds to (8,8), (7,7), (7,6), (6,5), (5,4), (4,3), (3,2), (2,1), (1,1), and (0,0).

Once we've finished, we reconstruct the alignment as follows: Starting with the last value, we reach (i,j) using the previously-calculated path. A diagonal jump implies there is an alignment (either a match or a mismatch). A top-down jump implies there is a deletion. A left-right jump implies there is an insertion.

For the example, we get:

Sequence 1 = A-CACACTA

Sequence 2 = AGCACAC-A

Motivation

One motivation for local alignment is the difficulty of obtaining correct alignments in regions of low similarity between distantly related biological sequences, because mutations have added too much 'noise' over evolutionary time to allow for a meaningful comparison of those regions. Local alignment avoids such regions altogether and focuses on those with a positive score, i.e. those with an evolutionary conserved signal of similarity. A prerequisite for local alignment is a negative expectation score. The expectation score is defined as the average score that the scoring system (substitution matrix and gap penalties) would yield for a random sequence.

Another motivation for using local alignments is that there is a reliable statistical model (developed by Karlin and Altschul) for optimal local alignments. The alignment of unrelated sequences tends to produce optimal local alignment scores which follow an extreme value distribution. This property allows programs to produce an expectation value for the optimal local alignment of two sequences, which is a measure of how often two unrelated sequences would produce an optimal local alignment whose score is greater than or equal to the observed score. Very low expectation values indicate that the two sequences in question might be homologous, meaning they might share a common ancestor.

However, the Smith-Waterman algorithm is fairly demanding of time and memory resources: in order to align two sequences of lengths m and n, $O(mn)$ time and space are required. As a result, it has largely been replaced in practical use by the BLAST algorithm; although not guaranteed to find optimal alignments, BLAST is much more efficient.

An implementation of the Smith-Waterman Algorithm, SSEARCH, is available in the FASTA sequence analysis package from. This implementation includes Altivec accelerated code for PowerPC G4 and G5 processors that speeds up comparisons 10- 20-fold, using a modification of the Wozniak, 1997 approach, and an SSE2 vectorization developed by Farrar making optimal protein database searches quite practical.

Accelerated Versions

FPGA

Cray demonstrated acceleration of the Smith-Waterman algorithm using a reconfigurable computing platform based on FPGA chips, with results showing up to 28x speed-up over standard microprocessor-based solutions.

Another FPGA based version of the Smith-Waterman algorithm shows FPGA (Virtex-4) speedups up to 100x over a 2.2 GHz Opteron processor. The TimeLogic DeCypher and CodeQuest systems also accelerate Smith-Waterman and Framesearch using PCIe FPGA cards.

Convey Computer Corporation's HC-1, an example of hybrid-core computing, has demonstrated a Smith-Waterman implementation that is 172x faster than SSEARCH in FASTA on a 3.0 GHz Intel Nehalem core with Farrar's implementation using the SSE2 instruction set. Over a more traditional software implementation it is a couple thousand times faster. The Convey result was obtained on a single Convey HC-1 server.

GPU

Recent work developed at Lawrence Livermore National Laboratory and the US Department of Energy's Joint Genome Institute accelerates Smith-Waterman local sequence alignment searches using graphics processing units (GPUs) with preliminary results showing a 2x speed-up over software implementations. A similar method has already been implemented in the Biofacet software since 1997, with the same speed-up factor.

Several GPU implementations of the algorithm in NVIDIA's CUDA C platform are also available. When compared to the best known CPU implementation (using SIMD instructions on the x86 architecture), by Farrar, the performance tests of this solution using a single NVidia GeForce 8800 GTX card show a slight increase in performance for smaller sequences, but a slight decrease in performance for larger ones. However the same tests running on dual NVidia GeForce 8800 GTX cards are almost twice as fast as the Farrar implementation for all sequence sizes tested.

A newer GPU CUDA implementation of SW is now available that is faster than previous versions and also removes limitations on query lengths.

Eleven different SW implementations on CUDA have been reported, three of which report speedups of 30X.

SSE

In 2000, a fast implementation of the Smith-Waterman algorithm using the SIMD technology available in Intel Pentium MMX processors and similar technology was described in a publication by Rognes and Seeberg.

In contrast to the Wozniak (1997) approach, the new implementation was based on vectors parallel with the query sequence, not diagonal vectors.

The company Sencel Bioinformatics has applied for a patent covering this approach. Sencel is developing the software further and provides executables for academic use free of charge.

A SSE2 vectorization of the algorithm (Farrar, 2007) is now available providing an 8-fold speedup on Intel/AMD processors with SSE2 extensions. When running on Intel processor using the Core microarchitecture the SSE2 implementation achieves a 20-fold increase.

Danish bioinformatics company CLC bio has achieved speed-ups of close to 200 over standard software implementations with SSE2 on a Intel 2.17 GHz Core 2 Duo CPU, according to a publicly available white paper.

Accelerated version of the Smith-Waterman algorithm, on Intel and AMD based Linux servers, is supported by the GenCore 6 package, offered by Biocceleration. Performance benchmarks of this software package show up to 10 fold speed acceleration relative to standard software implementation on the same processor.

Currently the only company in bioinformatics to offer both SSE and FPGA solutions accelerating Smith-Waterman, CLC bio has achieved speed-ups of more than 110 over standard software implementations with CLC Bioinformatics Cube.

Cell Broadband Engine

In 2008, Farrar described a port of the Striped Smith-Waterman to the Cell Broadband Engine and reported speeds of 32 and 12 GCUPS on an IBM QS20 blade and a Sony PlayStation 3, respectively.

Mathematical Optimal and Heuristic Methods

In mathematics, computer science and economics, optimization, or mathematical programming, refers to choosing the best element from some set of available alternatives.

In the simplest case, this means solving problems in which one seeks to minimize or maximize a real function by systematically choosing the values of real or integer variables from within an allowed set. This formulation, using a scalar, real-valued objective function, is probably the simplest example; the generalization of optimization theory and techniques to other formulations comprises a large area of applied mathematics. More generally, it means finding "best available" values of some objective function given a defined domain, including a variety of different types of objective functions and different types of domains.

History

The first optimization technique, which is known as steepest descent, goes back to Gauss. Historically, the first term to be introduced was "linear programming", which was due to George B. Dantzig, although much of the theory had been introduced by Leonid Kantorovich in 1939. Dantzig published the Simplex algorithm in 1947, and John von Neumann developed the theory of the duality in the same year. The term *programming* in this context does not refer to computer programming. Rather, the term comes from the use of *program* by the United States military to refer to proposed training and logistics schedules, which were the problems that Dantzig was studying at the time.

Other important mathematicians in the optimization field include:

- Richard Bellman
- Ronald A. Howard
- Leonid Kantorovich
- Narendra Karmarkar
- William Karush
- Leonid Khachiyan
- Bernard Koopman
- Harold Kuhn
- Joseph Louis Lagrange
- Laszlo Lovasz
- Arkadii Nemirovskii
- Yurii Nesterov
- John von Neumann
- Boris Polyak
- Lev Pontryagin
- James Renegar
- R. Tyrrell Rockafellar
- Cornelis Roos
- Naum Z. Shor
- Michael J. Todd
- Albert Tucker.

Major Subfields

- Convex programming studies the case when the objective function is convex and the constraints, if any, form a convex set. This can be viewed as a particular case of nonlinear programming or as generalization of linear or convex quadratic programming.

— Linear programming (LP), is a type of convex programming, studies the case in which the objective function f is linear and the set of constraints is specified using only linear equalities and inequalities. Such a set is called a polyhedron or a polytope if it is bounded.

— Second order cone programming (SOCP) is a convex program, and includes certain types of quadratic programs.

— Semidefinite programming (SDP) is a subfield of convex optimization where the underlying variables are semidefinite matrices. It is generalization of linear and convex quadratic programming.

— Conic programming is a general form of convex programming. LP, SOCP and SDP can all be viewed as conic programs with the appropriate type of cone.

— Geometric programming is a technique whereby objective and inequality constraints expressed as posynomials and equality constraints as monomials can be transformed into a convex program.

• Integer programming studies linear programs in which some or all variables are constrained to take on integer values. This is not convex, and in general much more difficult than regular linear programming.

• Quadratic programming allows the objective function to have quadratic terms, while the set A must be specified with linear equalities and inequalities. For specific forms of the quadratic term, this is a type of convex programming.

• Nonlinear programming studies the general case in which the objective function or the constraints or both contain nonlinear parts. This may or may not be a convex program. In general, the convexity of the program affects the difficulty of solving more than the linearity.

• Stochastic programming studies the case in which some of the constraints or parameters depend on random variables.

• Robust programming is, as stochastic programming, an attempt to capture uncertainty in the data underlying the optimization problem. This is not done through the use of random variables, but instead, the problem is solved taking into account inaccuracies in the input data.

- Combinatorial optimization is concerned with problems where the set of feasible solutions is discrete or can be reduced to a discrete one.
- Infinite-dimensional optimization studies the case when the set of feasible solutions is a subset of an infinite-dimensional space, such as a space of functions.
- Heuristic algorithms
  — Metaheuristics
- Constraint satisfaction studies the case in which the objective function f is constant (this is used in artificial intelligence, particularly in automated reasoning).
  — Constraint programming.
- Disjunctive programming used where at least one constraint must be satisfied but not all. Of particular use in scheduling.

In a number of subfields, the techniques are designed primarily for optimization in dynamic contexts (that is, decision making over time):

- Calculus of variations seeks to optimize an objective defined over many points in time, by considering how the objective function changes if there is a small change in the choice path.
- Optimal control theory is a generalization of the calculus of variations.
- Dynamic programming studies the case in which the optimization strategy is based on splitting the problem into smaller subproblems. The equation that describes the relationship between these subproblems is called the Bellman equation.
- Mathematical programming with equilibrium constraints is where the constraints include variational inequalities or complementarities.

Multi-objective Optimization

Adding more than one objective to an optimization problem adds complexity. For example, if you wanted to optimize a structural design, you would want a design that is both light and rigid. Because these two objectives conflict, a trade-off exists. There will be one lightest design, one stiffest design, and an infinite number of designs that are some compromise of weight and stiffness. This set of trade-off designs is known as a Pareto set. The curve created plotting weight against stiffness of the best designs is known as the Pareto frontier.

A design is judged to be Pareto optimal if it is not dominated by other designs: a Pareto optimal design must be better than another design in at least one aspect. If it is worse than another design in all respects, then it is dominated and is not Pareto optimal.

Multi-modal Optimization

Optimization problems are often multi-modal, that is they possess multiple good solutions. They could all be globally good (same cost function value) or there could be a mix of globally good and locally good solutions. Obtaining all (or at least some of) the multiple solutions is the goal of a multi-modal optimizer. Classical optimization techniques due to their iterative approach do not perform satisfactorily when they are used to obtain multiple solutions, since it is not guaranteed that different solutions will be obtained even with different starting points in multiple runs of the algorithm. Evolutionary Algorithms are however a very popular approach to obtain multiple solutions in a multi-modal optimization task.

Concepts and Notation

Optimization Problems

An optimization problem can be represented in the following way.

Given: a function $f : A \rightarrow R$ from some set A to the real numbers.

Sought: an element x_0 in A such that $f(x_0) \leq f(x)$ for all x in A ("minimization") or such that $f(x_0) \geq f(x)$ for all x in A ("maximization").

Such a formulation is called an optimization problem or a mathematical programming problem (a term not directly related to computer programming, but still in use for example in linear programming). Many real-world and theoretical problems may be modelled in this general framework. Problems formulated using this technique in the fields of physics and computer vision may refer to the technique as energy minimization, speaking of the value of the function f as representing the energy of the system being modelled.

Typically, A is some subset of the Euclidean space R^n, often specified by a set of *constraints*, equalities or inequalities that the members of A have to satisfy. The domain A of f is called the *search space* or the *choice set*, while the elements of A are called *candidate solutions* or *feasible solutions*. The function f is called, variously, an objective function, cost function, energy function, or energy functional. A feasible solution that minimizes (or maximizes, if that is the goal) the objective function is called an *optimal solution*.

Holds; that is to say, on some region around x^* all of the function values are greater than or equal to the value at that point. Local maxima are defined similarly. A large number of algorithms proposed for solving non-convex problems – including the majority of commercially available solvers – are not capable of making a distinction between local optimal solutions and rigorous optimal solutions, and will treat the former as actual solutions to the original problem.

The branch of applied mathematics and numerical analysis that is concerned with the development of deterministic algorithms that are capable of guaranteeing convergence in finite time to the actual optimal solution of a non-convex problem is called global optimization.

Classification of Critical Points and Extrema

Feasibility Problem

The satisfiability problem, also called the feasibility problem, is just the problem of finding any feasible solution at all without regard to objective value. This can be regarded as the special case of mathematical optimization where the objective value is the same for every solution, and thus any solution is optimal. Many optimization algorithms need to start from a feasible point. One way to obtain such a point is to relax the feasibility conditions using a slack variable; with enough slack, any starting point is feasible. Then, minimize that slack variable until slack is null or negative.

Existence

The extreme value theorem of Karl Weierstrass states that a continuous real-valued function on a compact set attains its maximum and minimum value. More generally, a lower semi-continous function on a compact set attains its minimum; an upper semi-continous function on a compact set attains its maximum.

Sufficient Conditions for Optimality

One of Fermat's theorems states that optima of unconstrained problems are found at stationary points, where the first derivative or the gradient of the objective function is zero. More generally, they may be found at critical points, where the first derivative or gradient of the objective function is zero or is undefined, or on the boundary of the choice set. An equation stating that the first derivative equals zero at an interior optimum is sometimes called a 'first-order condition'.

Optima of inequality-constrained problems are instead found by the Lagrange multiplier method. This method calculates a system of inequalities called the 'Karush–Kuhn–Tucker conditions' or 'complementary slackness conditions', which may then be used to calculate the optimum.

While the first derivative test identifies points that might be optima, this test does not distinguish a point which is a minimum from one that is a maximum or one that is neither.

When the objective function is twice differentiable, these cases can be distinguished by checking the second derivative or the matrix of second derivatives (called the Hessian matrix) in unconstrained problems, or a matrix of second derivatives of the objective function and the constraints called the bordered Hessian. The conditions that distinguish maxima and minima from other stationary points are sometimes called 'second-order conditions'.

Sensitivity and Stability of Optima

The envelope theorem describes how the value of an optimal solution changes when an underlying parameter changes.

The maximum theorem of Claude Berge (1963) describes the continuity of an optimal solution as a function of underlying parameters.

Calculus of Optimization

For unconstrained problems with twice-differentiable functions, some critical points can be found by finding the points where the gradient of the objective function is zero (that is, the stationary points). More generally, a zero subgradient certifies that a local minimum has been found for minimization problems with convex functions and other locally Lipschitz functions.

Further, critical points can be classified using the definiteness of the Hessian matrix: If the Hessian is *positive* definite at a critical point, then the point is a local minimum; if the Hessian matrix is negative definite, then the point is a local maximum; finally, if indefinite, then the point is some kind of saddle point.

Constrained problems can often be transformed into unconstrained problems with the help of Lagrange multipliers. Lagrangian relaxation also can also provide approximate solutions to difficult constrained problems.

When the objective function is convex, then any local minimum will also be a global minimum. There exist efficient numerical techniques for minimizing convex functions, such as interior-point methods.

Computational Optimization Techniques

To solve problems, researchers may use algorithms that terminate in a finite number of steps, or iterative methods that converge to a solution (on some specified class of problems), or heuristics that may provide approximate solutions to some problems (although their iterates need not converge).

Optimization Algorithms

- Simplex algorithm of George Dantzig: For linear programming. Extensions of the simplex algorithm exist for quadratic programming and for linear-fractional programming. The simplex algorithm has variants that are especially suited for network optimization.
- Combinatorial algorithms

Iterative Methods

For some nonlinear problems, the computational complexity of evaluating gradients and Hessians can be excessive. Some many problems of nonlinear programming, the iterative methods differ according to whether they evaluate Hessians, gradients, or only function values. While evaluating Hessians and gradients improves the rate of convergence of methods, such evaluations increase the computational cost of each iteration, so that users must select a balance.

- Methods that evaluate Hessians (or approximate Hessians, using finite differences):
- — Newton's method
- — Sequential quadratic programming: A method for small-medium scale constrained problems. Some versions can handle large-dimensional problems.

- Methods that evaluate gradients or approximate gradients using finite differences (or even subgradients):

  — *Quasi-Newton Methods:* Iterative methods for medium-large problems.

  — *Conjugate Gradient Methods:* Iterative methods for large problems. (In theory, these methods terminate in a finite number of steps with quadratic objective functions, but this finite termination is not observed in practice on finite-precision computers.)

  — *Interior Point Methods:* This is a large classs of methods for constrained optimization. Some interior-point methods use only (sub)gradient information, and others of which require the evaluation of Hessians.

  — *Gradient Descent (alternatively, "steepest descent" or "steepest ascent"):* A method of historical and theoretical interest, which has had renewed interest for find approximate solutions of enormous problems.

  — *Subgradient Methods:* An iterative method for large locally Lipschitz functions using generalized gradients. Following Boris T. Polyak, subgradient–projection methods are similar to conjugate–gradient methods.

  — *Bundle Method of Descent:* An iterative method for small–medium sized problems with locally Lipschitz functions, particularly for convex minimization problems. (Similar to conjugate gradient methods)

  — *Ellipsoid Method:* An iterative method for small problems with quasiconvex objective functions and of great theoretical interest, particularly in establishing the polynomial time complexity of some combinatorial optimization problems. It has similarities with Quasi-Newton methods.

  — *Reduced Gradient Method:* (Frank–Wolfe) for approximate minimization of specially structured problems with linear constraints, especially with traffic networks. For general unconstrained problems, this method reduces to the gradient method, which is regarded as obsolete (for almost all problems).

- Methods that evaluate only function values: If a problem is continuously differentiable, then gradients can be approximated using finite differences, in which case a gradient-based method can be used.

— Interpolation Methods: (Michael J. D. Powell).

Global Convergence

More generally, if the objective function is not a quadratic function, then many optimization methods use other methods to ensure that some subsequence of iterations converges to an optimal solution. The first and still popular method for ensuring convergence relies on-line searches, which optimize a function along one dimension. A second and increasingly popular method for ensuring convergence uses trust regions. Both line searches and trust regions are used in modern methods of non-differentiable optimization.

Heuristics

Besides (finitely terminating) algorithms and (convergent) iterative methods, there are heuristics that can provide approximate solutions to some optimization problems:

- Differential evolution
- Dynamic relaxation
- Genetic algorithms
- Hill climbing
- Nelder-Mead simplicial heuristic: A popular heuristic for approximate minimization (without calling gradients)
- Particle swarm optimization
- Simulated annealing
- Tabu search.

Applications

Problems in rigid body dynamics (in particular articulated rigid body dynamics) often require mathematical programming techniques, since you can view rigid body dynamics as attempting to solve an ordinary differential equation on a constraint manifold; the constraints are various nonlinear geometric constraints such as "these two points must always coincide", "this surface must not penetrate any other", or "this point must always lie somewhere on this curve". Also, the problem of computing contact forces can be done by solving a linear complementarity problem, which can also be viewed as a QP (quadratic programming) problem. Many design problems can also be expressed as optimization programs. This application is called design optimization. One subset is the engineering optimization, and another recent and growing subset of this field is multidisciplinary design optimization, which, while useful in many problems, has in particular been applied to aerospace engineering problems.

Economics also relies heavily on mathematical programming. An often studied problem in microeconomics, the utility maximization problem, and its dual problem the Expenditure minimization problem, are economic optimization problems. Consumers and firms are assumed to maximize their utility/profit.

Also, agents are most frequently assumed to be risk-averse thereby wishing to minimize whatever risk they might be exposed to. Asset prices are also explained using optimization though the underlying theory is more complicated than simple utility or profit optimization. Trade theory also uses optimization to explain trade patterns between nations. Another field that uses optimization techniques extensively is operations research.

Solvers

- Comet
- CPLEX
- FortSP-solver for stochastic programming problems
- Gurobi
- IMSL Numerical Libraries are collections of math and statistical algorithms available in C/C++, Fortran, Java and C#/.NET. Optimization routines in the IMSL Libraries include unconstrained, linearly and nonlinearly constrained minimizations, and linear programming algorithms.
- IPOPT-an open-source primal-dual interior point method NLP solver which handles sparse matrices
- KNITRO-solver for nonlinear optimization problems
- MATLAB Optimization Toolbox-solvers for linear and nonlinear optimization problems
- Mathematica-handles linear programming, integer programming and constrained non-linear optimization problems
- Merlin-A Fortran-77, user friendly open source software package, for non-linear optimization with bound constraints.

- MINUIT
- NAG Libraries-local and global optimization routines available for multiple programming languages (C, C++, Fortran, Python, Java, .NET, GPUs), packages (MATLAB, Maple, Excel) and for SMP and multicore
- OpenOpt-a free optimization framework written in Python and NumPy, connects to tens of solvers, can involve Automatic differentiation
- NLopt a free optimization library, callable from C/C++/Fortran/Python/Scheme, which interfaces to a large number algorithms for global and local constrained and unconstrained nonlinear optimization.
- Opt++-An object-oriented package from Lawrence Berkeley and Sandia National Labs, used for nonlinear optimization.
- SNOPT
- SmartDO Engineering design optimization package.

Chapter 6

Bioinformatics Databases

What is a Database?

A database consists of an organized collection of data for one or more uses, typically in digital form. One way of classifying databases involves the type of their contents, for example: bibliographic, document-text, statistical. Digital databases are managed using database management systems, which store database contents, allowing data creation and maintenance, and search and other access.

Architecture

Database architecture consists of three levels, *external*, *conceptual* and *internal*. Clearly separating the three levels was a major feature of the relational database model that dominates 21st century databases.

The external level defines how users understand the organization of the data. A single database can have any number of views at the external level. The internal level defines how the data is physically stored and processed by the computing system. Internal architecture is concerned with cost, performance, scalability and other operational matters. The conceptual is a level of indirection between internal and external. It provides a common view of the database that is uncomplicated by details of how the data is stored or managed, and that can unify the various external views into a coherent whole.

Database Management Systems

A database management system (DBMS) consists of software that operates databases, providing storage, access, security, backup and other facilities. Database management systems can be categorized according to the database model that they support, such as relational or XML, the type(s) of computer they support, such as a server cluster or a mobile phone, the query language(s) that access the database, such as SQL or XQuery, performance trade-offs, such as maximum scale or maximum speed or others. Some DBMS cover more than one entry in these categories, e.g., supporting multiple query languages. Examples of some commonly used DBMS are MySQL, PostgreSQL, Microsoft Access, SQL Server, FileMaker,Oracle, Sybase, dBASE, Clipper, FoxPro etc. Almost every database software comes with an Open Database Connectivity (ODBC) driver that allows the database to integrate with other databases.

Components of DBMS

Most DBMS as of 2009 implement a relational model. Other DBMS systems, such as Object DBMS, offer specific features for more specialized requirements. Their components are similar, but not identical.

RDBMS Components

- Sublanguages— Relational DBMS (RDBMS) include Data Definition Language (DDL) for defining the structure of the database, Data Control Language (DCL) for defining security/access controls, and Data Manipulation Language (DML) for querying and updating data.
- Interface drivers—These drivers are code libraries that provide methods to prepare statements, execute statements, fetch results, etc. Examples include ODBC, JDBC, MySQL/PHP, FireBird/Python.
- SQL engine—This component interprets and executes the DDL, DCL, and DML statements. It includes three major components (compiler, optimizer, and executor).
- Transaction engine—Ensures that multiple SQL statements either succeed or fail as a group, according to application dictates.
- Relational engine—Relational objects such as Table, Index, and Referential integrity constraints are implemented in this component.
- Storage engine—This component stores and retrieves data from secondary storage, as well as managing transaction commit and rollback, backup and recovery, etc.

ODBMS Components

Object DBMS (ODBMS) has transaction and storage components that are analogous to those in an RDBMS. Some DBMS handle DDL,

DML and update tasks differently. Instead of using sublanguages, they provide APIs for these purposes. They typically include a sublanguage and accompanying engine for processing queries with interpretive statements analogous to but not the same as SQL. Example object query languages are OQL, LINQ, JDOQL, JPAQL and others. The query engine returns collections of objects instead of relational rows.

Types

Operational Database: These databases store detailed data about the operations of an organization. They are typically organized by subject matter, process relatively high volumes of updates using transactions. Essentially every major organization on earth uses such databases. Examples include customer databases that record contact, credit, and demographic information about a business' customers, personnel databases that hold information such as salary, benefits, skills data about employees, Enterprise resource planning that record details about product components, parts inventory, and financial databases that keep track of the organization's money, accounting and financial dealings.

Data Warehouse: Data warehouses archive modern data from operational databases and often from external sources such as market research firms. Often operational data undergoes transformation on its way into the warehouse, getting summarized, anonymized, reclassified, etc. The warehouse becomes the central source of data for use by managers and other end-users who may not have access to operational data.

For example, sales data might be aggregated to weekly totals and converted from internal product codes to use UPC codes so that it can be compared with ACNielsen data.Some basic and essential components of data warehousing include retrieving and analysing data, transforming,loading and managing data so as to make it available for further use.

Analytical Database: Analysts may do their work directly against, a data warehouse, or create a separate analytic database for *Online Analytical Processing.* For example, a company might extract sales records for analysing the effectiveness of advertising and other sales promotions at an aggregate level.

Distributed Database: These are databases of local work-groups and departments at regional offices, branch offices, manufacturing plants and other work sites. These databases can include segments of both common operational and common user databases, as well as data generated and used only at a user's own site.

End-user Database: These databases consist of data developed by individual end-users. Examples of these are collections of documents in spreadsheets, word processing and downloaded files, even managing their personal baseball card collection.

External Database: These databases contain data collected for use across multiple organizations, either freely or via subscription. The Internet Movie Database is one example.

Hypermedia Databases: The Worldwide web can be thought of as a database, albeit one spread across millions of independent computing systems. Web browsers "process" this data one page at a time, while web crawlers and other software provide the equivalent of database indexes to support search and other activities.

Models

Post-relational Database Models

Products offering a more general data model than the relational model are sometimes classified as post-relational. Alternate terms include "hybrid database", "Object-enhanced RDBMS" and others. The data model in such products incorporates relations but is not constrained by E.F. Codd's Information Principle, which requires that all information in the database must be cast explicitly in terms of values in relations and in no other way.

Some of these extensions to the relational model integrate concepts from technologies that pre-date the relational model. For example, they allow representation of a directed graph with trees on the nodes.

Some post-relational products extend relational systems with non-relational features. Others arrived in much the same place by adding relational features to pre-relational systems. Paradoxically, this allows products that are historically pre-relational, such as PICK and MUMPS, to make a plausible claim to be post-relational.

Object Database Models

In recent years, the object-oriented paradigm has been applied in areas such as engineering and spatial databases, telecommunications and in various scientific domains. The conglomeration of object oriented programming and database technology led to this new kind of database.

These databases attempt to bring the database world and the application-programming world closer together, in particular by ensuring that the database uses the same type system as the application program. This aims to avoid the overhead (sometimes referred to as the *impedance mismatch*) of converting information between its representation in the database and its representation in the application program (typically as objects). At the same time, object databases attempt to introduce key ideas of object programming, such as encapsulation and polymorphism, into the world of databases.

A variety of these ways have been tried for storing objects in a database. Some products have approached the problem from the application-programming side, by making the objects manipulated by the program persistent. This also typically requires the addition of some kind of query language, since conventional programming languages do not provide language-level functionality for finding objects based on their information content. Others have attacked the problem from the database end, by defining an object-oriented data model for the database, and defining a database programming language that allows full programming capabilities as well as traditional query facilities.

Storage Structures

Databases may store relational tables/indexes in memory or on hard disk in one of many forms:

- ordered/unordered flat files
- ISAM
- heaps
- hash buckets
- logically-blocked files
- B+ trees.

The most commonly used are B+ trees and ISAM.

Object databases use a range of storage mechanisms. Some use virtual memory-mapped files to make the native language (C++, Java etc.) objects persistent. This can be highly efficient but it can make multi-language access more difficult. Others disassemble objects into fixed-and varying-length components that are then clustered in fixed sized blocks on disk and reassembled into the appropriate format on either the client or server address space. Another popular technique involves storing the objects in tuples (much like a relational database) which the database server then reassembles into objects for the client.

Other techniques include clustering by category (such as grouping data by month, or location), storing pre-computed query results, known as materialized views, partitioning data by range (e.g., a data range) or by hash.

Memory management and storage topology can be important design choices for database designers as well. Just as normalization is used to reduce storage requirements and improve database designs, conversely denormalization is often used to reduce join complexity and reduce query execution time.

Indexing

Indexing is a technique for improving database performance. The many types of index share the common property that they eliminate the need to examine every entry when running a query. In large databases, this can reduce query time/cost by orders of magnitude. The simplest form of index is a sorted list of values that can be searched using a binary search with an adjacent reference to the location of the entry, analogous to the index in the back of a book. The same data can have multiple indexes (an employee database could be indexed by last name and hire date.)

Indexes affect performance, but not results. Database designers can add or remove indexes without changing application logic, reducing maintenance costs as the database grows and database usage evolves.

Given a particular query, the DBMS' query optimizer is responsible for devising the most efficient strategy for finding matching data. The optimizer decides which index or indexes to use, how to combine data from different parts of the database, how to provide data in the order requested, etc.

Indexes can speed up data access, but they consume space in the database, and must be updated each time the data is altered. Indexes therefore can speed data access but slow data maintenance. These two properties determine whether a given index is worth the cost.

Transactions

As every software system, a DBMS operates in a faulty computing environment and prone to failures of many kinds. A failure can corrupt the respective database unless special measures are taken to prevent this. A DBMS achieves certain levels of fault tolerance by encapsulating in database transactions units of work (executed programs) performed upon the respective database.

The Acid Rules

Most DBMS provide some form of support for transactions, which allow multiple data items to be updated in a consistent fashion, such that updates that are part of a transaction succeed or fail in unison. The so-called ACID rules, summarized here, characterize this Behaviour:

- Atomicity: Either all the data changes in a transaction must happen, or none of them. The transaction must be completed, or else it must be undone (rolled back).

- Consistency: Every transaction must preserve the declared consistency rules for the database.

- Isolation: Two concurrent transactions cannot interfere with one another. Intermediate results within one transaction must remain invisible to other transactions. The most extreme form of isolation is serializability, meaning that transactions that take place concurrently could instead be performed in some series, without affecting the ultimate result.

- Durability: Completed transactions cannot be aborted later or their results discarded. They must persist through (for instance) DBMS restarts.

In practice, many DBMSs allow the selective relaxation of these rules to balance perfect Behaviour with optimum performance.

Concurrency Control and Locking

Concurrency control is essential for the correctness of transactions executed concurrently in a DBMS, which is the common execution mode for performance reasons. The main concern and goal of concurrency control is isolation.

Isolation

Isolation refers to the ability of one transaction to see the results of other transactions. Greater isolation typically reduces performance and/or concurrency, leading DBMSs to provide administrative options to reduce isolation. For example, in a database that analyses trends rather than looking at low-level detail, increased performance might justify allowing readers to see uncommitted changes ("dirty reads".)

A common way to achieve isolation is by locking. When a transaction modifies a resource, the DBMS stops other transactions from also modifying it, typically by locking it. Locks also provide one method of ensuring that data does not change while a transaction is reading it or even that it doesn't change until a transaction that once read it has completed.

Lock Types

Locks can be *shared* or *exclusive*, and can lock out *readers* and/ or *writers*. Locks can be created *implicitly* by the DBMS when a transaction performs an operation, or *explicitly* at the transaction's request. Shared locks allow multiple transactions to lock the same resource. The lock persists until all such transactions complete. Exclusive locks are held by a single transaction and prevent other transactions from locking the same resource.

Read locks are usually shared, and prevent other transactions from modifying the resource. Write locks are exclusive, and prevent other transactions from modifying the resource. On some systems, write locks also prevent other transactions from reading the resource.

The DBMS implicitly locks data when it is updated, and may also do so when it is read. Transactions explicitly lock data to ensure that they can complete without complications. Explicit locks may be useful for some administrative tasks.

Locking can significantly affect database performance, especially with large and complex transactions in highly concurrent environments.

Lock Granularity

Locks can be coarse, covering an entire database, fine-grained, covering a single data item, or intermediate covering a collection of data such as all the rows in a RDBMS table.

Deadlocks

Deadlocks occur when two transactions each require data that the other has already locked exclusively. Deadlock detection is performed by the DBMS, which then aborts one of the transactions and allows the other to complete.

Replication

Database replication involves maintaining multiple copies of a database on different computers, to allow more users to access it, or to allow a secondary site to immediately take over if the primary site stops working. Some DBMS piggyback replication on top of their transaction logging facility, applying the primary's log to the secondary in near real-time. Database clustering is a related concept for handling larger databases and user communities by employing a cluster of multiple computers to host a single database that can use replication as part of its approach.

Security

Database security denotes the system, processes, and procedures that protect a database from unauthorized activity.

DBMSs usually enforce security through access control, auditing, and encryption:

- Access control manages who can connect to the database via authentication and what they can do via authorization.
- Auditing records information about database activity: who, what, when, and possibly where.
- Encryption protects data at the lowest possible level by storing and possibly transmitting data in an unreadable form. The DBMS encrypts data when it is added to the database and decrypts it when returning query results. This process can occur on the client side of a network connection to prevent unauthorized access at the point of use.

Confidentiality

Law and regulation governs the release of information from some databases, protecting medical history, driving records, telephone logs, etc.

In the United Kingdom, database privacy regulation falls under the Office of the Information Commissioner. Organizations based in the United Kingdom and holding personal data in digital format such as databases must register with the Office.

Different Types of Biological Databases

Biological databases are libraries of life sciences information, collected from scientific experiments, published literature, high-throughput experiment technology, and computational analyses. They contain information from research areas including genomics, proteomics, metabolomics, microarray gene expression, and phylogenetics. Information contained in biological databases includes gene function, structure, localization (both cellular and chromosomal), clinical effects of mutations as well as similarities of biological sequences and structures.

Relational database concepts of computer science and Information retrieval concepts of digital libraries are important for understanding biological databases. Biological database design, development, and long-term management is a core area of the discipline of bioinformatics. Data contents include gene sequences, textual descriptions, attributes and ontology classifications, citations, and tabular data. These are often described as semi-structured data, and can be represented as tables, key delimited records, and XML structures. Cross-references among databases are common, using database accession numbers.

Overview

Biological databases are an important tool in assisting scientists to understand and explain a host of biological phenomena from the structure of biomolecules and their interaction, to the whole metabolism of organisms and to understanding the evolution of species. This knowledge helps facilitate the fight against diseases, assists in the development of medications and in discovering basic relationships amongst species in the history of life.

Biological knowledge is distributed amongst many different general and specialized databases. This sometimes makes it difficult to ensure the consistency of information. Biological databases cross-reference other databases with accession numbers as one way of linking their related knowledge together.

An important resource for finding biological databases is a special yearly issue of the journal *Nucleic Acids Research* (NAR). The Database Issue of NAR is freely available, and categorizes many of the publicly available online databases related to biology and bioinformatics.

Output

Biological data comes in many formats. These formats include text, sequence data, protein structure and links. Each of these can be found from certain sources, for example:

- Text formats are provided by PubMed and OMIM.
- Sequence data are provide by GenBank, in terms of DNA, and UniProt, in terms of protein.
- Protein structures are provided by PDB, SCOP, and CATH.

Problems Associated with Protein Databases

Since discovery in the area of protein structure has not evolved quite as quickly as discoveries in the area sequence data, due to the 3D nature of protein structure, less information is available for it.

Nonetheless, data can be accessed through members of the wwPDB (PDBe, PDBj and RCSB PDB, SCOP-Structural Classification of Proteins- at ([1]), and CATH at (]).

Species-specific Databases

Species-specific databases are available for some species, mainly those that are often used in research. For example, Colibase ([3]) is an *E. coli* database. Other popular species specific databases include, Flybase ([4]) for *Drosophila*, and WormBase ([5]) for the nematodes *Caenorhabditis elegans* and *Caenorhabditis briggsae*.

List of Biological Databases

Primary Sequence Databases

The International Nucleotide Sequence Database (INSD) consists of the following databases.

1. DDBJ (DNA Data Bank of Japan)
2. EMBL Nucleotide Sequence DB (European Molecular Biology Laboratory)
3. GenBank (National Centre for Biotechnology Information).

The three databases, DDBJ (Japan), GenBank (USA) and EMBL Nucleotide Sequence Database (Europe), are repositories for nucleotide sequence data from all organisms.

All three databases accept nucleotide sequence submissions, and then exchange new and updated data on a daily basis to achieve optimal synchronisation between them. These three databases are primary databases, as they house original sequence data.

Metadatabases

Strictly speaking a metadatabase can be considered a database of databases, rather than any one integration project or technology. They collect data from different sources and usually make them available in new and more convenient form, or with an emphasis on a particular disease or organism.

1. Entrez (National Centre for Biotechnology Information)
2. euGenes (Indiana University)
3. GeneCards (Weizmann Inst.)
4. SOURCE (Stanford University)
5. mGen containing four of the world biggest databases GenBank, Refseq, EMBL and DDBJ-easy and simple program friendly gene extraction
6. Bioinformatic Harvester (Karlsruhe Institute of Technology)- Integrating 26 major protein/gene resources.
7. MetaBase (KOBIC)-A user contributed database of biological databases.
8. ConsensusPathDB-A molecular functional interaction database, integrating information from 12 other databases.

Genome Databases

These databases collect organism genome sequences, annotate and analyse them, and provide public access. Some add curation of experimental literature to improve computed annotations. These databases may hold many species genomes, or a single model organism genome.

1. CAMERA Resource for microbial genomics and metagenomics
2. Corn, the Maize Genetics and Genomics Database
3. EcoCyc a database that describes the genome and the biochemical machinery of the model organism *E. coli K-12*
4. Ensembl provides automatic annotation databases for human, mouse, other vertebrate and eukaryote genomes.
5. PATRIC, the PathoSystems Resource Integration Centre
6. Flybase, genome of the model organism Drosophila melanogaster
7. MGI Mouse Genome (Jackson Lab.)
8. JGI Genomes of the DOE-Joint Genome Institute provides databases of many eukaryote and microbial genomes.
9. National Microbial Pathogen Data Resource. A manually curated database of annotated genome data for the pathogens Campylobacter, Chlamydia, Chlamydophila, Haemophilus, Listeria, Mycoplasma, Neisseria, Staphylococcus, Streptococcus, Treponema, Ureaplasma, and Vibrio.

10. Saccharomyces Genome Database, genome of the yeast model organism.

11. Viral Bioinformatics Resource Centre Curated database containing annotated genome data for eleven virus families.

12. The SEED platform for microbial genome analysis includes all complete microbial genomes, and most partial genomes. The platform is used to annotate microbial genomes using subsystems.

13. Xenbase, genome of the model organism Xenopus tropicalis and Xenopus laevis

14. Wormbase, genome of the model organism Caenorhabditis elegans

15. Zebrafish Information Network, genome of this fish model organism.

16. TAIR, The Arabidopsis Information Resource.

17. UCSC Malaria Genome Browser, genome of malaria causing species (*Plasmodium falciparumata* and others)

18. RGD Rat Genome Database: Genomic and phenotype data for Rattus norvegicus

Protein Sequence Databases

1. UniProt Universal Protein Resource (UniProt Consortium: EBI, Expasy, PIR)

2. PIR Protein Information Resource (Georgetown University Medical Centre (GUMC))

3. Swiss-Prot Protein Knowledgebase (Swiss Institute of Bioinformatics)

4. Pedant Protein Extraction, Description and ANalysis Tool (Forschungszentrum f. Umwelt & Gesundheit)

5. Prosite Database of Protein Families and Domains

6. DIP Database of Interacting Proteins (Univ. of California)

7. Pfam Protein families database of alignments and HMMs (Sanger Institute)

8. Prints Prints is a compendium of protein fingerprints (Manchester University)

9. ProDom Comprehensive set of Protein Domain Families (INRA/ CNRS)

10. SignalP 3.0 Server for signal peptide prediction (including cleavage site prediction), based on artificial neural networks and HMMs

11. Superfamily Library of HMMs representing superfamilies and database of (superfamily and family) annotations for all completely sequenced organisms

12. Annotation Clearing House a project from the National Microbial Pathogen Data Resource.

Protein Structure Databases

1. Protein Data Bank (PDB) (Research Collaboratory for Structural Bioinformatics (RCSB))

2. SCOP Structural Classification of Proteins

3. CATH Protein Structure Classification.

Protein Model Databases

1. SWISS-MODEL Server and Repository for Protein Structure Models

2. ModBase Database of Comparative Protein Structure Models (Sali Lab, UCSF)

3. Protein Model Portal (PMP) Meta database that combines several databases of protein structure models (Biozentrum, Basel, Switzerland).

Carbohydrate Structure Databases

1. EuroCarbDB, A repository for both carbohydrate sequences/ structures and experimental data.

Protein-protein Interactions

1. BioGRID A General Repository for Interaction Datasets (Samuel Lunenfeld Research Institute)

2. String: String is a database of known and predicted protein-protein interactions. (EMBL)

3. DIP Database of Interacting Proteins

4. BIND Biomolecular Interaction Network Database

5. NetPro

Signalling Pathway Databases

- Netpath-A curated resource of signal transduction pathways in humans

- Reactome
- NCI-Nature Pathway Interaction Database
- SignaLink Database

Metabolic Pathway Databases

1. BioCyc Database Collection including EcoCyc and MetaCyc
2. Kegg Pathway Database (Univ. of Kyoto)
3. Manet database (University of Illinois)
4. Reactome(Cold Spring Harbour Laboratory, EBI, Gene Ontology Consortium).

Microarray Databases

The term microarray database is usually used to describe a repository containing microarray gene expression data. The key features of a microarray database are to store the measurement data, manage a searchable index, and make the data available to other applications for analysis and interpretation (either directly, or via user downloads).

Microarray databases can fall into two distinct classes:

1. A peer reviewed, public repository that adheres to academic or industry standards and is designed to be used by many analysis applications and groups. A good example of this is the Gene Expression Omnibus (GEO) from NCBI or ArrayExpress from EBI.

2. A specialized repository associated primarily with the brand of a particular entity (lab, company, university, consortium, group), an application suite, a topic, or an analysis method, whether it is commercial, non-profit, or academic. These databases might have one or more of the following characteristics:

   — A subscription or license may be needed to gain full access,

   — The content may come primarily from a specific group (e.g. SMD, or UPSC-BASE),

   — There may be constraints on who can use the data or for what purpose data can be used,

   — Special permission may be required to submit new data, or there may be no obvious process at all,

— Only certain applications may be equipped to use the data, often also associated with the same entity (for example, caArray at NCI is specialized for the caBIG),

— Further processing or reformatting of the data may be required for standard applications or analysis,

— They claim to address the 'urgent need' to have a standard, centralized repository for microarray data.,

— There is a claim to an incremental improvement over one of the public repositories,

— A meta-analysis *application*, which incorporates studies from one or more public databases (e.g. Gemma primarily uses GEO studies; NextBio uses various sources)

1. ArrayExpress (European Bioinformatics Institute)
2. Gene Expression Omnibus (National Centre for Biotechnology Information)
3. GPX(Scottish Centre for Genomic Technology and Informatics)
4. maxd (Univ. of Manchester)
5. Stanford Microarray Database (SMD) (Stanford University).

Mathematical Model Databases

1. Biomodels Database
2. CellML

PCR/Real Time PCR Primer Databases

1. PathoOligoDB: A free QPCR oligo database for pathogens.

Specialized Databases

- Antibody Central Antibody information database and search resource.
- BIOMOVIE (ETH Zurich) movies related to biology and biotechnology
- CGAP Cancer Genes (National Cancer Institute)
- Clone Registry Clone Collections (National Centre for Biotechnology Information)
- Connectivity map Transcriptional expression data and correlation tools for drugs

- CTD The Comparative Toxicogenomics Database describes chemical-gene-disease interactions
- DBGET H.sapiens (Univ. of Kyoto)
- DiProDB A database to collect and analyse thermodynamic, structural and other dinucleotide properties.
- Dryad a repository of data underlying scientific publications in evolution, ecology, and related fields
- Edinburgh Mouse Atlas
- GreenPhylDB (A phylogenomic database for plant comparative genomics)
- GDB Hum. Genome Db (Human Genome Organisation)
- HGMD disease-causing mutations (HGMD Human Gene Mutation Database)
- HUGO (Official Human Genome Database: HUGO Gene Nomenclature Committee)
- HvrBase++ Human and primate mitochondrial DNA
- Interferome The Database of Interferon Regulated Genes
- List with SNP-Databases
- NCBI-UniGene (National Centre for Biotechnology Information)
- Oncogenomic databases A compilation of databases that serve for cancer research.
- OMIM Inherited Diseases (Online Mendelian Inheritance in Man)
- OrthoMaM (A database of Orthologous Mammalian Markers)
- p53 The p53 Knowledgebase
- PhenCode linking human mutations with phenotype
- Plasma Proteome Database Human plasma proteins along with their isoforms
- PolygenicPathways Genes and risk factors implicated in Alzheimer's disease, Bipolar disorder, Autism or Schizophrenia, multiple sclerosis and Parkinson's disease
- SHMPD The Singapore Human Mutation and Polymorphism Database
- SciClyc An Open-access database to shared antibodies, cell cultures, and documents for biomedical research.

- SNPSTR database A database of SNPSTRs-compound genetic markers consisting of a microsatellite (STR) and one tightly linked SNP-in human, mouse, rat, dog and chicken.
- TreeBASE An open-access database of phylogenetic trees and the data behind them
- XTractor Discovering Newer Scientific Relations Across PubMed Abstracts. A tool to obtain manually annotated relationships for Proteins, Diseases, Drugs and Biological Processes as they get published in PubMed.

Biobank

A biobank is a cryogenic storage facility used to archive biological samples for use in research and experiments. Ranging in size from individual refrigerators to warehouses, biobanks are maintained by institutions such as hospitals, universities, nonprofit organizations, and pharmaceutical companies.

Security and Storage

Biobanks, like other DNA databases, must carefully store and document access to samples and donor information. The samples must be maintained reliably with minimal deterioration over time, and they must be protected from physical damage, both accidental and intentional. The registration of each sample entering and exiting the system is centrally stored, usually on a computer-based system that can be backed up frequently.

The physical location of each sample is noted to allow the rapid location of specimens. Archival systems de-identify samples to respect the privacy of donors and allow blinding of researchers to analysis. The database, including clinical data, is kept separately with a secure method to link clinical information to tissue samples. Room temperature storage of samples is sometimes used, and was developed in response to perceived disadvantages of low-temperature storage, such as costs and potential for freezer failure. Current systems are small and are capable of storing nearly 40,000 samples in about one tenth of the space required by a -80 °C $(-112$°F) freezer. Replicates or split samples are often stored in separate locations for security.

One controversy of large databases of genetic material is the question of ownership of samples. To date, Iceland has had three different laws on ownership of the physical samples and the information they contain. Current Icelandic law holds that the Icelandic government has custodial rights of the physical samples themselves while the donors retain ownership rights. In contrast, Tonga and Estonia give ownership of biobank samples to the government, but their laws include strong protections of donor rights.

Gene Bank

Gene banks help preserve genetic material, be it plant or animal. In plants, this could be by freezing cuts from the plant, or stocking the seeds. In animals, this is the freezing of sperm and eggs in zoological freezers until further need. With corals, fragments are taken which are stored in water tanks under controlled conditions.

In plants, it is possible to unfreeze the material and propagate it, however, in animals, a living female is required for artificial insemination. While it is often difficult to utilize frozen animal sperm and eggs, there are many examples of it being done successfully.

In an effort to conserve agricultural biodiversity, gene banks are used to store and conserve the plant genetic resources of major crop plants and their crop wild relatives. There are many gene banks all over the world, with the Svalbard Global Seed Vault being probably the most famous one.

NCBI

The National Centre for Biotechnology Information (NCBI) is part of the United States National Library of Medicine (NLM), a branch of the National Institutes of Health. The NCBI is located in Bethesda, Maryland (38°592 423 N 77°052 583 W 38.994994°N 77.099339°W/38.994994; -77.099339; Coordinates: 38°592 423 N 77°052 583 W/ 38.994994°N 77.099339°/38.994994; -77.099339) and was founded in 1988 through legislation sponsored by Senator Claude Pepper. The NCBI houses genome sequencing data in GenBank and an index of biomedical research articles in PubMed Central and PubMed, as well as other information relevant to biotechnology. All these databases are available online through the Entrez search engine.

NCBI is directed by David Lipman, one of the original authors of the BLAST sequence alignment program and a widely respected figure in Bioinformatics. He also leads an intramural research program, including groups led by Stephen Altschul (another BLAST co-author), David Landsman, and Eugene Koonin (a prolific author on comparative genomics).

GenBank

The NCBI has had responsibility for making available the GenBank DNA sequence database since 1992. GenBank coordinates with individual laboratories and other sequence databases such as those of the European Molecular Biology Laboratory (EMBL) and the DNA Data Bank of Japan (DDBJ).

Since 1992, NCBI has grown to provide other databases in addition to GenBank. NCBI provides Online Mendelian Inheritance in Man, the Molecular Modelling Database (3D protein structures), dbSNP a database of single-nucleotide polymorphisms, the Unique Human Gene Sequence Collection, a Gene Map of the human genome, a Taxonomy Browser, and coordinates with the National Cancer Institute to provide the Cancer Genome Anatomy Project. The NCBI assigns a unique identifier (Taxonomy ID number) to each species of organism.

The NCBI has software tools that are available by WWW browsing or by FTP. For example, BLAST is a sequence similarity searching program. BLAST can do sequence comparisons against the GenBank DNA database in less than 15 seconds.

NCBI Bookshelf

The NCBI Bookshelf is a collection of freely available, downloadable, on-line versions of selected biomedical books. As of March 2006, the Bookshelf had 55 titles covering aspects of molecular biology, biochemistry, cell biology, genetics, microbiology, a couple of disease states from a molecular and cellular point of view, research methods, and virology. Some of the books are online versions of previously published books, while others, such as Coffee Break (book), are written and edited by NCBI staff. The Bookshelf is a complement to the Entrez PubMed repository of peer-reviewed publication abstracts in that Bookshelf contents provide established perspectives on evolving areas of study and a context in which many disparate individual pieces of reported research can be organized.

DbSNP

The Single Nucleotide Polymorphism Database (dbSNP) is a free public archive for genetic variation within and across different species developed and hosted by the National Centre for Biotechnology Information (NCBI) in collaboration with the National Human Genome Research Institute (NHGRI). Although the name of the database implies a collection of one class of polymorphisms only (i.e., single nucleotide polymorphisms (SNPs)), it in fact contains a range of molecular variation:

(1) SNPs,

(2) short deletion and insertion polymorphisms (indels/DIPs),

(3) microsatellite markers or short tandem repeats (STRs),

(4) multinucleotide polymorphisms (MNPs),

(5) heterozygous sequences, and

(6) named variants.

The dbSNP accepts apparently neutral polymorphisms, polymorphisms corresponding to known phenotypes, and regions of no variation. It was created in September 1998 to supplement GenBank, NCBI's collection of publicly available nucleic acid and protein sequences.

As of build 131 (available February 2010), dbSNP had amassed over 184 million submissions representing more than 64 million distinct variants for 55 organisms, including *Homo sapiens*, *Mus musculus*, *Oryza sativa*, and many other species.

Purpose

DbSNP is an online resource implemented to aid biology researchers. Its goal is to act as a single database that contains all identified genetic variation, which can be used to investigate a wide variety of genetically based natural phenomenon.

Specifically, access to the molecular variation cataloged within dbSNP aids basic research such as physical mapping, population genetics, investigations into evolutionary relationships, as well as being able to quickly and easily quantify the amount of variation at a given site of interest. In addition, dbSNP guides applied research in pharmacogenomics and the association of genetic variation with phenotypic traits. According to the NCBI website, "The long-term investment in such novel and exciting research [dbSNP] promises not only to advance human biology but to revolutionise the practice of modern medicine."

Submission

Source: dbSNP accepts submissions for any organism from a wide variety of sources including individual research laboratories, collaborative polymorphism discovery efforts, large scale genome sequencing centres, other SNP databases (e.g. the SNP consortium, HapMap, etc.), and private businesses.

2. Types of Records

Every submitted variation receives a submitted SNP ID number ("ss#"). This accession number is a stable and unique identifier for that submission. Unique submitted SNP records also receive a reference SNP ID number ("rs#"; "refSNP cluster"). However, more than one record of a variation will likely be submitted to dbSNP, especially for clinically relevant variations. To accommodate this, dbSNP routinely assembles identical submitted SNP records into a single reference SNP record, which is also a unique and stable identifier.

3. How to Submit

To submit variations to dbSNP, one must first acquire a submitter handle, which identifies the laboratory responsible for the submission. Next, the author is required to complete a submission file containing the relevant information and data. Submitted records must contain the ten essential pieces of information listed in the following table.

Other information required for submissions includes contact information, publication information (title, journal, authors, year), molecule type (genomic DNA, cDNA, mitochondrial DNA, chloroplast DNA), and organism.

Element	*Explanation*
Flanking DNA	Variations from assays must have 25 bp of flanking sequence on either side of the polymorphism and must be 100 bp overall.
Alleles	Alleles must be defined using A, G, C, or T nomenclature; IUPAC nomenclature will only be accepted in flanking regions.
Method	A description of how the variation was detected (e.g. DNA sequencing) or how the allele frequencies were calculated. A table of method classes is provided.
Population	A description of the initial group from which the variation was found or from which the allele frequency was calculated. A table of population classes is provided.

Contd...

Element	*Explanation*
Sample size	The number of chromosomes used to find the variation and the number of chromosomes used to calculate allele frequencies.
Population-specific allele frequency	The allele frequency of the surveyed population.
Population-specific genotype frequency	The genotype frequency of the surveyed population.
Population-specific heterozygosity	The proportion of individuals who are heterozygous for the variation.
Individual genotypes	The genotype of individuals from the study.
Validation information	The validation status lists the categories of evidence supporting the variation.

Release

New information obtained by dbSNP becomes available to the public periodically in a series of "builds" (i.e. revisions and releases of data). There is no schedule for releasing new builds; instead, builds are usually released when a new genome build becomes available, assuming that the genome has some cataloged variation associated with it.

This occurs approximately every 1–2 months. Genome sequences often contain errors so reference SNPs ("refSNP") from previous builds, as well as new submitted SNPs, are re-mapped to the newly available genome sequence through multiple cycles of BLAST and MegaBLAST.

Multiple submitted SNPs, if mapping to the same location, are clustered into one refSNP cluster and are assigned a reference SNP ID number. However, if two refSNP cluster records are found to map to the same location (i.e. are identical), then dbSNP will also merge those records together.

In this case, the smallest refSNP number ID (i.e. the earliest record) would now represent both records, and the larger refSNP number IDs would become obsolete. These obsolete refSNP number IDs and are not used again for new records. When a merger of two refSNP records occurs, the change is tracked, and the former refSNP number IDs can still be used as a search query.

This process of merging identical records together reduces redundancy within dbSNP.

There are two exceptions to the above merging criteria. First, if there exists two classes of variation at one site (e.g. a SNP and a DIP), then the two refSNP number IDs are not merged. Secondly, clinically important refSNPs that have been cited in the literature are termed "precious" and are never merged so as to prevent later confusion.

Retrieval

How to: The dbSNP can be searched using the Entrez SNP search tool. A variety of queries can be used for searching: an ss number ID, a refSNP number ID, a gene name, an experimental method, a population class, a population detail, a publication, a marker, an allele, a chromosome, a base position, a heterozygosity range, a build number, or a strain. In addition, many results can be retrieved simultaneously using batch queries. Searches return refSNP number IDs that match the query term and a summary of the available information for that refSNP cluster.

Tools/Data: The information available for a refSNP cluster includes the basic information from each of the individual submissions as well as information available from combining the data from multiple submissions (e.g. heterozygosiity, genotype frequencies). Many tools are available to examine a refSNP cluster in greater depth. Map view shows the position of the variation in the genome and other nearby variations. Another tool, gene view reports the location of the variation within a gene (if it is in a gene), the old and new codon, the amino acids encoded by both, and whether the change is synonymous or non-synonymous. Sequence viewer shows the position of the variant in relation to introns, exons, and other distant and close variants. 3D structure mapping, which shows 3D images of the encoded protein is also available.

The dbSNP is also linked to many other NCBI resources including the nucleotide, protein, gene, taxonomy and structure databases, as well as pubmed, Uni STS, PMC, OMIM, and Uni Gene.

Validation Status: The validation status list the categories of evidence that support a variant. These include: (1) multiple independent submissions; (2) frequency or genotype data; (3) submitter confirmation;

(4) observation of all alleles in at least two chromosomes; (5) genotyped by HapMap; and (6) sequenced in the 1000 Genomes Project.

Problems

The quality of the data found on dbSNP has been questioned by many research groups, which suspect high false positive rates due to genotyping and base-calling errors. These mistakes can easily be entered into dbSNP if the submitter uses (1) uncritical bioinformatic alignments of highly similar but distinct DNA sequences, and/or (2) PCRs with primers that cannot discriminate between similar but distinct DNA sequences. Mitchell *et al.* (2004) reviewed four studies and concluded that dbSNP has a false positive rate between 15-17% for SNPs, and also that the minor allele frequency is greater than 10% for approximately 80% of the SNPs that are not false positives. Similarly, Musemeci *et al.* (2010) states that as many as 8.32% of the biallelic coding SNPs in dbSNP are artifacts of highly similar DNA sequences (i.e. paralogous genes) and refer to these entries as single nucleotide differences (SNDs).

The high error rates in dbSNP may not be surprising: of the 23.7 million refSNP entries for humans, only 14.5 million have been validated, leaving the remaining 9.2 million as candidate SNPs. However, according to Musemeci *et al.* (2010), even the validation code provided in the refSNP record is only partially useful: only HapMap validation reduced the number of SNDs (3% vs 8%), but only accepting this method removes more than half of the real SNPs in the dbSNP. These authors also note that one source of submissions from the Lee group are plagued with errors: 20% of these submissions are SNDs (vs. 8% for submissions). However, as the authors note, ignoring all of these submissions would remove many real SNPs.

Errors in the dbSNP can hamper candidate gene association studies and haplotype-based investigations. Errors may also increase false conclusions in association studies: increasing the number of SNPs that are tested by testing false SNPs requires more hypothesis tests. However, these false SNPs cannot actually be associated with traits, so the alpha level is decreased more than is necessary for a rigorous test if only the true SNPs were tested and the false negative rate will increase. Musemeci *et al.* (2010) suggested that authors of negative association studies inspect their previous studies for false SNPs (SNDs), which could be removed from analysis.

PubMed

PubMed is a free database accessing the Medline database of citations, abstracts and some full text articles on life sciences and biomedical topics. The United States National Library of Medicine (NLM) at the National Institutes of Health (NIH) maintains PubMed as part of the Entrez information retrieval system. Listing an article or journal in PubMed is not endorsement. In addition to Medline, PubMed also offers access to:

- Oldmedline for pre-1966 citations. This has recently been enhanced, and records for 1951+, even those parts in the printed indexes, are now included within the main portion.

- Citations to all articles (even those that are out-of-scope, e.g., covering plate tectonics or astrophysics) from certain Medline journals, primarily the most important general science and chemistry journals, from which the life sciences articles are indexed for Medline.

- In-process citations which provide a record for an article before it is indexed with MeSH and added to Medline or converted to out-of-scope status (Premedline).

- Citations that precede the date that a journal was selected for Medline indexing (when supplied electronically by the publisher).

- Some life science journals that submit full text to the PubMed Central digital library and may not have been recommended for inclusion in Medline although they have undergone a review by NLM, and some physics journals that were part of a prototype PubMed in the early to mid-1990s.

Many PubMed citations contain links to full text articles which are freely available, often in PubMed Central. In late 2007, President George W. Bush signed the Consolidated Appropriations Act of 2007 (H.R. 2764) into law; this law included a provision requiring the NIH to modify its policies and require inclusion into PubMed Central complete electronic copies of their peer-reviewed research and findings from its funded research. This is the first time the US government has required an agency to provide open access to research and is an evolution from the 2005 policy, in which the NIH asked researchers to voluntarily add their research to PubMed Central. With an effective date of 7 April 2008, the Department of Health and Human Services gave notice: "The Director of the National Institutes of Health shall require that all investigators funded by the NIH submit or have submitted for them to the National Library of Medicine's PubMed Central an electronic version of their final, peer-reviewed manuscripts upon acceptance for publication, to be made publicly available no later than 12 months after the official date of publication: Provided, That the NIH shall implement the public access policy in a manner consistent with copyright law".

The National Library of Medicine also leases the Medline information to a number of private vendors such as Ovid and SilverPlatter – as well as many other vendors. PubMed was first released in January 1996..

Information about the journals indexed in PubMed is found in its Journals Database, searchable by subject or journal title, Title Abbreviation, the NLM ID (NLM's unique journal identifier), the ISO abbreviation, and both the print and electronic International Standard Serial Numbers (pISSN and eISSN). The database includes all journals in all Entrez databases.

As of 27 October 2010 (2010 -10-27), PubMed has over 20 million citations going back to 1966, and selectively to the year 1865, and *very* selectively to 1809. Some 11.5 million articles are listed with their abstract and 3.1 million articles are available full-text for free, either from the publisher or as part of PubMed's PMC collection.

Searching PubMed

PMID

A PMID (PubMed identifier or PubMed unique identifier) is a unique number assigned to each PubMed citation of life sciences and biomedical scientific journal articles. The related Pubmed Central archive may additionally assign a separate number, a PMCID (PubMed Central identifier), normally written with a PMC prefix.

As of 2005, there are roughly between 15 and 16 million PMID numbers in use, starting from 1, and about 1 million new numbers are added each year. 'Unique identifier' (UID) is the search field tag used in the PubMed search query.

The assignment of a PMID or PMCID to a publication tells the reader nothing about the type or quality of the content. PMIDs are assigned to letters to the editor, editorial opinions, op-ed columns, and any other piece that the editor chooses to include in the journal, as well as peer-reviewed papers. The existence of the identification number is also not proof that the papers have not been retracted for fraud, incompetence, or misconduct. The announcement about any corrections to original papers may be assigned a PMID.

Comprehensive Search

For comprehensive, optimal searching in PubMed, it is necessary to have a thorough understanding of its core component, Medline, and especially of the MeSH (Medical Subject Headings) controlled vocabulary used to index Medline articles.

The new PubMed interface, launched in October 2009, encourages the use of quick, Google-like search formulations:

Quick Search

Quick, simple telegram-style search formulations can also be used, and they generally produce acceptable results. PubMed automatically links textwords to relevant MeSH terms. Aspects of the question can then be added successively, in a Google-like fashion, until a number of 'hits' judged manageable is achieved. No knowledge of actual MeSH terms, Boolean operators, English or American spelling, 'nesting', or record-fields is required. PubMed's intelligent search algorithm does (or implies) this in the background. Examples of such simple telegram-style questions and results they produce on PubMed:

- Question 1: Optimal management of radial head fractures? Randomized controlled trials?

Telegram-style question in PubMed search window: radial head fractures randomized

Result: 9 records found, one judged highly relevant.

- Question 2: Paper by Glasziou on radial fractures in the BMJ in 2007?

Telegram-style question in PubMed search window: glasziou fractures bmj 2007

Result: 1 record (the target) found.

- Question 3: State of vitreous body (of the eye) and time of death? A review, perhaps?

Telegram-style question in PubMed search window: vitreous body time death review.

Result: 8 records found, several relevant, e.g. Madea/Rödig (2006).

Clinical Queries/Systematic Reviews

A special feature of PubMed is the 'Clinical Queries' and 'Systematic Reviews' option which can be used to identify more relevant (robust) studies by automatically applying study-type 'filters' to a search. This feature was updated and re-designed in June 2010.

Related Articles

After a quick search, references which are judged particularly relevant can be marked and 'related articles' can be identified. If relevant, several studies can be selected and 'related articles' to all of them can be generated.

The 'related articles' are then listed on order or 'relatedness' (not chronological order). To create the list of 'related articles' PubMed compares words from the Title and Abstract of each citation, as well as the MeSH headings assigned, using a powerful word-weighted algorithm.

Mapping to MeSH (Headings) and Subheadings

A strong feature of PubMed is its ability to automatically link to Medical Subject Headings (MeSH) and Subheadings. Examples would be: 'bad breath' links to (and includes in the search) 'Halitosis', 'Writers cramp' to 'focal dystonia', 'breast cancer' to 'breast neoplasms'. Where appropriate, these MeSH terms are automatically 'expanded'. Terms like 'nursing' are automatically linked to 'Nursing [Mesh]' or 'Nursing [Subheading]'. This important feature makes PubMed searches automatically more sensitive and avoids false-negative (missed) hits by compensating for the diversity of medical terminology.

Searching with Tags and Boolean Operators

Tags: Field names/tags are not normally required in a search formulation. For example:

> *pnas drexler ke 1981*
>
> *will yield a single reference, and is the equivalent (in this example) of*
>
> *pnas [ta] AND drexler ke[au] AND 1981[dp]*
>
> *For strings of characters which may appear in different fields the field tag has to be added, for example:*
>
> *1981[pg] pnas*

> *correctly identifies a few article starting on page 1981 in PNAS.*
>
> *green[ti] green[au]*
>
> *will identify a few papers by an author named Green with the word 'green' in the title.*

Some of the most common Tags/Field Names are:

- [au] — author—e.g., Miller RA [au] or miller ra [au] (not case sensitive)
- [dp] — date published—e.g., 1998 [dp] or 1998/11/06 (YYYY/ MM/DD, where MM/DD are optional)
- [ip] — issue, part or supplement—e.g., 4 [ip] (for issue four of a volume)
- [la] — language—e.g., eng [la] (to only find articles in English)
- [page] — first page number of the article—e.g., 673 [pg] (for an article starting on page 673)
- [pmid] — PubMed ID—e.g., 15094092 [pmid] (to find the PubMed article with ID 15094092)
- [pt] — publication type—e.g., review [pt]
- [ta] — journal title—e.g., rejuvenation res [ta] (all articles in the journal Rejuvenation Research)
- [ti] — title words—e.g., endothelial [ti] (all articles with "endothelial" in the title)
- [vol] — volume—e.g., 101 [vol] (for volume number 101).

It should be noted that using field qualifiers automatically disables PubMed's 'mapping' function.

Boolean Operators

There are three Boolean operators: AND (intersection); OR (union); NOT (exclusion). NOT should be used with care as it may generate 'false-negative' results. The AND operator is assumed by default.

All Boolean operators are processed in a left-to-right sequence. The order in which PubMed processes a search statement can be specified by enclosing concepts in parentheses.

The terms inside the parentheses are processed first as a unit and then incorporated into the overall strategy.

For example:

dogs OR cats AND spleen

will correctly identify some 4,300 papers.

Spleen AND cats OR dogs

will incorrectly find some 120,000 articles.

Spleen AND (cats OR dogs) is correct.

If in doubt brackets should be used when 'mixing' Boolean operators.

Alternative Interfaces

The new PubMed interface, launched in October 2009, with its simple search window, encourages focused search formulations (instead of complex search strategies) when appropriate. It may disourage use of some of the alternative interfaces listed below which offered this simple search option at their opening search page.

- eTBLAST-a natural language text similarity engine for MEDLINE and other text databases.
- GoPubMed-Explore PubMed/MEDLINE with Gene Ontology (GO) and Medical Subject Headings (MeSH)
- HighWire Press-a medical search engine created by an online journal publishing house that searches within its collection of journals.
- HubMed-An alternative interface to the PubMed medical literature database.
- Pubget-Based on PubMed/MEDLINE but gets to the PDF right away, provided the journal is available for free or the subscription is being paid for.
- Quertle-A free, semantic-based search engine for PubMed, full-text articles, NIH Grants, TOXLINE, and news.

Interactome

Interactome is defined as the whole set of molecular interactions in cells. It is usually displayed as a directed graph. Molecular interactions can occur between molecules belonging to different biochemical families (proteins, nucleic acids, lipids, carbohydrates, etc.) and also within a given family. When spoken in terms of proteomics, interactome refers to protein-protein interaction network(PPI), or protein interaction network (PIN). Another extensively studied type of interactome is the protein-DNA interactome (network formed by transcription factors (and DNA or chromatin regulatory proteins) and their target genes. The word "interactome" was originally coined in 1999 by a group of French scientists headed by Bernard Jacq.

It has been suggested that the size of an organism's interactome correlates better than genome size with the biological complexity of the organism (Stumpf, et al., 2008). Although protein-protein interaction maps containing several thousands of binary interactions are now available for several organisms, none of them is presently complete and the size of interactomes is still a matter of debate. In 2010, the most "complete" gene interactome produced to date was compiled from 54 million two-gene comparisons to describe "the interaction profiles for ~75% of all genes in the Budding yeast," with 170,000 gene interactions.

Although extremely important and useful, the interactome is still being developed and is not complete (as of October 2010). There are various factors that have a role in protein interactions that have yet to be incorporated in the interactome. Many have termed the interactome as a whole as being fuzzy.

The binding strength of the various proteins, microenvironmental factors, sensitivity to various procedures, and the physiological state of the cell all affect protein-protein interactions, yet are not accounted for in the interactome. Although the interactome is useful in some ways, it must be analysed knowing that these factors exist and can affect the protein interactions.

Methods of Mapping the Interactome

The study of the interactome is called interactomics. The basic unit of protein network is protein-protein interaction (PPI). Because the interactome considers the whole organism, there is a need to collect a massive amount of information.

Experimental methods have been devised to determine PPI, such as affinity purification and yeast two hybrid (Y2H). The former is suited to identify a protein complex, while the latter is suited to explore the binary interactions in mass quantities. The former is considered as a low-throughput method (LTP), while the latter is considered as high-throughput method (HTP). Using the experimental data as a starting point, the concept of homology transfer has been used to develop algorithms to map the interactome, including ones that produce detailed atomic models of protein protein complexes as well as other protein-molecule interactions.

There have been several efforts to map the eukaryotic interactome through HTP methods. As of 2006, yeast, fly, worm, and human HTP maps have been created. Recently, pathogen-host interactome (Hepatitis C Virus/Human (2008), Epstein Barr virus/Human (2008), Influenza virus/Human (2009)) was also delineated through HTP to identify essential molecular components for pathoghens but also for the host to recognize pathogens and trigger efficient innate immune response.

Using the Interactome

Researchers have begun to use preliminary versions of the interactome to gain understanding about the biology and function of the molecules within them. For example, protein interaction networks have been used to produce improved protein functional annotations (or nannotations) for proteins with unknown functions.

MetaBase

MetaBase is a user-contributed database of biological databases, listing all the biological databases currently available on the internet. The initial release of MetaBase was derived entirely from the content of the Nucleic Acids Research (NAR) 2007 Database Issue. MetaBase is a wiki, using MediaWiki software as well as the Semantic MediaWiki extension.

MetaBase was developed as part of the BioWiki initiative, and was entered into the first International Openfree Bioinformation Contents Competition organised by BiO.CC, the top-level biological information web site operated by KOBIC.

Currently MetaBase contains details about nearly 1000 biological databases and over 800 'web services' derived from NAR, as well as more than 50 'user-contributed' databases.

Quertle

Quertle is a semantic search engine for life and chemical science literature and information. It covers a wide variety of information sources and, according to the company, is used by researchers in more than 150 countries.

How Quertle Works

Quertle uses semantic-based linguistics to automatically extract Subject Verb Object relationships asserted by the author(s) of each document. The identification of these assertions uses several methods including natural language processing. For full-text documents, Quertle includes only the main content, not, for example, the references.

The Subject Verb Object relationships are stored in a metadatabase and the user's query is matched against that metadata. This identifies documents based on meaning and context and generally provides fewer, but more relevant, hits than a traditional keyword search. Thus, Quertle is fundamentally different from search sites such as PubMed. Nonetheless, Quertle does simultaneously search a keyword index to find documents based on inclusion of the search terms. These are presented on a separate tab in the results.

An ontology covering genes, proteins, chemicals, diseases, cell types, and other life, chemical, and biomedical science nomenclature is used to automatically search for all variants of a term in the user's query. For example, a search for "aspirin" will find asserted relationships that mention "acetylsalicylic acid". The ontology also is used to find members of a class of entities, such as "neurotransmitters".

Content

Quertle indexes Medline, full-text articles from BioMed Central and PubMed Central (open access subset), NIH grants, the US National Library of Medicine Torex database, and biomedical news.

Snpstr

A SNPSTR is a compound genetic marker composed of one or more SNPs and one microsatellite (STR). SNPSTRs were first described by MOUNTAIN et al. (2002) who developed experimental protocols for autosomal SNPSTRs which contain a SNP and a microsatellite within 500 base pairs of one another. More recently a database that contains all SNPSTRs in five model genomes, including human, has been created.

Usage and Importance

There has been widespread and growing interest in genetic markers suitable for drawing population genetic inferences about past demographic events and to detect the effects of selection. Single nucleotide polymorphisms (SNPs) and microsatellites (or short tandem repeats, STRs) have received great attention in the analysis of human population history, even though they have both disadvantages. It was thus suggested that the combination of these two markers could give rise to better conclusions.

Database Similarity Searches

The terms, Similarity, Identity, and Homology each have a distinct meaning. Orthology and Paralogy are important concepts describing the relationship of members of a given protein family in one organism to the members of the same family in other organisms. (Reeck, G. R., de Haen, C. et al. (1987)).

General Approach

The General approach involves the use of a set of algorithms such as the BLAST programs to compare a query sequence to all the sequences in a specified database. Comparisons are made in a pairwise fashion. Each comparison is given a score reflecting the degree of similarity between the query and the sequence being compared. The higher the score, the greater the degree of similarity.

The similarity is measured and shown by aligning two sequences. Alignments can be global or local (algorithm specific). A global alignment is an optimal alignment that includes all characters from each sequence, whereas a local alignment is an optimal alignment that includes only the most similar local region or regions. Discriminating between real and artifactual matches is done using an estimate of probability that the match might occur by chance. Of course, similarity, by itself, cannot be considered a sufficient indicator of function.

The BLAST Algorithm

The BLAST programs (Basic Local Alignment Search Tools) are a set of sequence comparison algorithms introduced in 1990 that are used to search sequence databases for optimal local alignments to a query. The BLAST programs improved the overall speed of searches while retaining good sensitivity (important as databases continue to grow) by breaking the query and database sequences into fragments ("words"), and initially seeking matches between fragments. The initial search is done for a word of length "W" that scores at least "T" when compared to the query using a given substitution matrix. Word hits are then extended in either direction in an attempt to generate an alignment with a score exceeding the threshold of "S". The "T" parameter dictates the speed and sensitivity of the search.

Quantification

The quality of each pair-wise alignment is represented as a score and the scores are ranked. Scoring matrices are used to calculate the score of the alignment base by base (DNA) or amino acid by amino acid (protein). A unitary matrix is used for DNA pairs because each position can be given a score of +1 if it matches and a score of zero if it does not. Substitution matrices are used for amino acid alignments. These are matrices in which each possible residue substitution is given a score reflecting the probability that it is related to the corresponding residue in the query. The alignment score will be the sum of the scores for each position. Various scoring systems (e.g. PAM, BLOSUM and PSSM) for quantifying the relationships between residues have been used.

Gaps

Positions at which a letter is paired with a null are called gaps. Gap scores are negative. Since a single mutational event may cause the insertion or deletion of more than one residue, the presence of a gap is frequently ascribed more significance than the length of the gap. Hence the gap is penalized heavily, whereas a lesser penalty is assigned to each subsequent residue in the gap. There is no widely accepted theory for selecting gap costs. It is rarely necessary to change gap values from the default.

Significance

The significance of each alignment is computed as a P value or an E value. Each alignment must be viewed by a critical human eye before being accepted as meaningful. For example high scoring pairs whose similarity is based on repeated amino acid stretches (e.g. poly glutamine) are unlikely to reflect meaningful similarity between the query and the match. Filters, (e.g. SEG) that mask low complexity regions, can be applied to partially alleviate this problem.

Databases

A variety of DNA and protein databases are available. A protein database is appropriate for searches with an amino acid sequence as query. A nucleic acid database is generally appropriate for searches with a DNA query sequence. The exception to this occurs when using programs such as BLASTX and TBLASTN, which perform cross-comparisons between different types of query and database sequences. With genome sequencing projects producing huge amounts of sequence data, database sequence similarity search has become a central tool in bioinformatics to identify potentially homologous sequences.

It is thus widely used as an initial step for sequence characterization and annotation, phylogeny, genomics, transcriptomics, and proteomics studies. Database similarity search is based upon sequence alignment methods also used in pairwise sequence comparison. Sequence alignment can be global (whole sequence alignment) or local (partial sequence alignment) and there are algorithms to find the optimal alignment given particular comparison criteria.

However, as database searches require the comparison of the query sequence with every single sequence in the database, heuristic algorithms have been designed to reduce the time required to build an alignment that has a reasonable chance to be the best one.

Such algorithms have been implemented as fast and efficient programs (Blast, FastA) available in different types to address different kinds of problems. After searching the appropriate database, similarity search programs produce a list of similar sequences and local alignments.

These results should be carefully examined before coming to any conclusion, as many traps await the similarity seeker: paralogues, multidomain proteins, pseudogenes, etc.

This chapter presents points that should always be kept in mind when performing database similarity searches for various goals. It ends with a practical example of sequence characterization from a single protein database search using Blast.

Sqlj and Sql Plus

SQLJ is an ISO standard (ISO/IEC 9075-10) for embedding SQL statements in Java programs.

Whereas JDBC provides an API, SQLJ consists of a language extension. Thus programs containing SQLJ must be run through a preprocessor (the SQLJ translator) before they can be compiled.

Some advantages of SQLJ over JDBC include:

- SQLJ commands tend to be shorter than equivalent JDBC programs.
- SQL syntax can be checked at compile time.
- Preprocessor might generate static SQL which performs better than dynamic SQL because query plan is created on program compile time, stored in database and reused at runtime. Static SQL can guarantee worst case reply time and access plan stability. IBM DB2 supports static SQL use in SQLJ programs.

Disadvantages include:

- SQLJ requires a preprocessing step.
- Many IDEs do not have SQLJ support.
- SQLJ lacks support for most of the common persistence frameworks, such as Hibernate.

SQL*Plus

SQL*Plus is an Oracle command-line utility program that can run SQL and PL/SQL commands interactively or from a script.

SQL*Plus operates as a relatively simple tool with a basic command-line interface. Programmers and DBAs commonly use it as the default available fundamental interface in almost any Oracle software installation.

Command Types

SQL*Plus understands three categories of text:

1. SQL statements
2. PL/SQL blocks
3. SQL*Plus internal commands, for example:
   — environment control commands such as SET
   — environment monitoring commands such as SHOW

Scripts can include all of these components.

An Oracle programmer in the appropriately-configured software environment can launch SQL*Plus, for example, by entering:

sqlplus scott/tiger

Where the Oracle user scott has the password tiger. SQL*Plus then presents a prompt with the default form of:

SQL>

Interactive use can then start by entering a SQL statement (terminated by a semicolon), a PL/SQL block, or another command.

History

The first version of SQL*Plus was called *UFI* ("User Friendly Interface"). UFI appeared in Oracle database releases up to Version 4.

After Oracle programmers had added new features to UFI, its name became *Advanced UFI*. The name "Advanced UFI" changed to "SQL*Plus" before the release of this version.

As of 2010 the product continues to bear the name *SQL*Plus*.

Usage

Graphical interfaces from Oracle or third parties have diminished the proportion of Oracle database end-users who depend on the SQL*Plus environment. Oracle shops typically continue to use SQL*Plus scripts for batch updating or simple reports. Oracle Corporation's wrappers/gui-fications/replacements for SQL*Plus include:

- Oracle SQL*Plus Worksheet, a component of OEM
- iSQL*Plus or iSQLPlus, a web-based utility
- SQL Worksheet, a component of Oracle SQL Developer
- SQL Workshop (part of Oracle Application Express).

Oracle 11g

Starting from Oracle database 11g, iSqlplus (web based) and sqlplus graphical GUI no longer ship with Oracle database software. The command-line SQL*Plus interface continues in use, mostly for non-interactive scripting or for administrative purposes (connect internal before Oracle 8i; sqlplus... as sysdba later).

Compatibility

Other vendors have made their software somewhat compatible with SQL*Plus script commands or offer a SQL*Plus mode of operation. Relevant products include TOAD from Quest Software.

Integration

Variables: SQL*Plus-internal variables, accessible within an SQL*Plus session, include:

- user variables, displayable with the DEFINE command and referenceable with one or two cases of a prefixed character (default prefixes: '&' and '&&')
  — predefined variables, prefixed with an underscore ('_')
  — substitution variables, useful for interacting with user-input
- bind variables, prefixed by a colon (':'), which can interact with the PL/SQL environment. Displayable with the Variable and Print commands.

Supplementary Software

- SQL Assistant SQL Assistant add-on for SQL*Plus Windows version extends SQL*Plus with SQL automatic word completion, in-line Oracle SQL Reference, data export/import, code unit testing, data browsing, and code development functions.
- rlwrap rlwrap does GNU Readline like command completion for SQL*Plus on UNIX and Linux.

Internet based Biological Databases

Bioinformatics is critically dependent upon computer science and related technologies. Benton [BEN, 1996] states, "Bioinformatics stands on the foundations of computational science and engineering, and applied mathematics, and depends on large stores of both experimental and derived data." Benton describes many computer technologies and their interrelationship to bioinformatics applications.

Both software and hardware play critical roles in bioinformatics. "The amount of information available is growing exponentially. This has been largely because of an increasing sophistication in cloning and sequencing techniques, but also because of the ever increasing development of computing software and hardware coupled with decreasing costs" [SAN, 2000].

Processing Power

Perhaps the most important computer-related factor that has contributed to the growth of bioinformatics has been the increase in computer processing power coupled with decreasing costs. Inexpensive, powerful data processing makes tasks such as complex biological algorithmic computations possible. Powerful microprocessors can influence bioinformatics in other ways too. "Arguably, it was only Intel's development of the Pentium microprocessor that allowed Applied Biosystems and Amersham Pharmacia to create DNA sequencing machines capable of unravelling the genome 4 years ahead of original forecasts" [STOK, 2001].

The application of tremendous processing power to biological computations is clearly shown in the example of IBM's Blue Gene supercomputer. "Twelve to fifteen times more powerful than today's top supercomputer, Blue Gene houses a million processors, each capable of performing a billion operations per second... Blue Gene's first assignment will be to tackle one of biology's toughest computational problems: Predicting the structure of a protein from its building blocks — complicated strings of amino acids that contain thousands of atoms. When these molecules are formed in a cell, they fold themselves into exactly the right configuration in a matter of seconds. But with large proteins, no existing computer is powerful enough to predict the exact pattern of folds" [LIC, 2001].

Networks

The growth of networks, networking standards, and the Internet have had revolutionarily effects on the sharing of data and knowledge and thus have had a profound effect on bioinformatics, a field focused on biological data acquisition, management, and analysis. The TCP/IP networking standard was developed in the 1970's and was incorporated into Berkeley Software Distribution (BSD) UNIX, version 4.2, after which time it became the networking protocol standard for the Internet.

Open networking standards play a critical role in access to data over networks. Previous to the establishment of the TCP/IP standard, computerized network communication could be exceedingly difficult, since lower-level network programming could be required in order for communication to proceed.

An alternative to open standards is to use proprietary networking packages such as CICS, but this ties network communications to proprietary technology and can be platform-dependent. As an example of the problems of lacking a networking protocol standard, the planning of the Distributed INGRES database system was greatly hindered by the lack of UNIX networking software, which didn't appear until BSD 4.2. The TCP/IP-based Internet and in particular the World Wide Web have made a staggering amount of biological data available. The graphical nature of the Web allows for data exchange in a straightforward, easy-to-use manner. This is very useful for biologists who may not be versed in some of the more esoteric computer communication methods designed by computer scientists for computer scientists.

Network programming technologies have been developed that allow for flexible and powerful distributed bioinformatics applications. Programming via sockets has been a complicated way of writing network applications, although Java socket programming is relatively easy compared to socket programming in C/C++. CORBA (Common Object Request Broker Architecture) and Microsoft's DCOM (Distributed Component Object Model) are powerful but complex standards for distributed computing. Java RMI offers a way of writing distributed applications in a fairly simple manner. Java RMI is similar to CORBA, but limits the implementation language to Java. Other Java technologies such as applets and servlets offer new ways to program across networks. These topics will be investigated in greater detail in the "Distributed Computing Paradigms" section.

Databases

The maturation of database technology has been an essential reason for the growth of bioinformatics. Modern database management systems (DBMSs) are capable of managing vast quantities of data and handling complex operations such as concurrency control and recovery management in an efficient manner. Relational databases are well understood and standardized.

Object-oriented databases lack the standardization of relational databases but allow for the storage of complex objects under the control of the DBMS. External objects can also be saved in relational databases, for instance, as an Oracle BLOB (binary large object) data type. Object-relational databases extend the relational model to have object-oriented features.

Database concepts such as indices can be used for rapid retrieval of biological data. Decreasing memory prices can lead to faster query processing, since increased memory allows for significant database data buffering, which avoids excessive query processing slowdown due to I/O. Celera's database was essential in the storage and analysis of their human genome sequence data. Data warehousing and database federations are techniques that play important roles in biological data integration.

Relational Databases

Relational databases are the most predominant type of database used today. The relational database model was proposed by Dr. E.F. Codd in 1970. This model consists of a group of relations, operators to operate on those relations, and integrity constraints. A relation is a two-dimensional table that stores data, and a relational database contains one or more tables.

A row in a table is known as a tuple or a record, and it represents a data set concerning a particular entity. A column represents a particular attribute of an entity, and a field occurs where a row and column intersect. A primary key is a column or group of columns that can   uniquely identify each tuple in a table. It is possible to relate data in different tables through the use of foreign keys. A foreign key is a column or group of columns that refers to the primary key in another table or even the same table.

SQL (Structured Query Language) is the standard query language used to query and manage data in a database. The Select statement is used for retrieving data. The DML (data manipulation language) statements of SQL are Insert, Update, and DELETE, and these are used to insert, modify, and remove rows from database tables. The transaction control statements are Commit, Savepoint, and Rollback. These statements are used to govern database transactions. The DDL (data definition language) statements are Alter, Create, Drop, Rename, and Truncate, and they allow for tasks such as creating and removing tables. The DCL (data control language) statements are GRANT and Revoke, and they are responsible for controlling database access rights.

The first attribute is ID, which is a unique identification number for each sequence entry in the table. The ID attribute would be the primary key of the table, since it uniquely identifies each row. The next attribute is Description, which offers a verbal description of the entry. The Organism attribute indicates what species the sequence comes from, and the SEQUENCE attribute contains the actual sequence of nucleic acids. The '...' entries in the table indicate additional characters are present but not shown.

Data in the table can easily be queried using the SQL Select statement, as in the following example:

Select Organism

From sequence_table

Where ID='hsighaf';

This Select statement would select the organism attribute from the table from the rows in which the ID attribute is equal to the given alphanumeric identification number listed on the Where line. This query would generate the following response:

Organism

Homo sapiens

As another example, we could ask the database for all the IDs for sequences that begin with 'a':

Select ID

From sequence_table

Where sequence like 'a%';

This would generate the response:

ID

TRBG361

MM12341

Databases used by the data integration system are typically queried via web servers using CGI programs or other similar technologies.

In this imaginary query, a CGI program called getorganism is executed with the query string MM12341 on the web server at mybiodatabase. The purpose of this program is to retrieve the organism specified by the ID number MM12341. If the program is a C++ program, it might use an ODBC driver to query the database using a SQL query such as:

Select organism

From sequence_table

Where ID='MM12341';

The CGI program can obtain the result of the query and then return this result to the user, possibly formatted in HTML for viewing in a web browser.

Thus, if the database being queried is a relational database, although a query such as a call to a CGI program may not resemble a SQL query, the underlying actual access of the database may involve a SQL query.

Sequence Databases

In the field of bioinformatics, a sequence database is a large collection of computerized ("digital") nucleic acid sequences, protein sequences, or other sequences stored on a computer. A database can include sequences from only one organism (e.g., a database for all proteins in Saccharomyces cerevisiae), or it can include sequences from all organisms whose DNA has been sequenced.

Search Issues

Sequence databases can be searched using a variety of methods. The most common is probably searching for a sequence similar to a certain target protein or gene whose sequence is already known to the user. The BLAST program is a method of this type.

Many Inputs Create Inconsistencies

A major problem with all the large genetic sequence databases is that records are deposited in them from a wide range of sources, from individual researchers to large genome sequencing centres.

As a result, the sequences themselves, and especially the biological annotations attached to these sequences, vary tremendously in quality. Also there is much redundancy, as multiple labs often submit numerous sequences that are identical, or nearly identical, to others in the databases.

Many annotations are based not on laboratory experiments, but on the results of sequence similarity searches for previously-annotated sequences. Of course, once a sequence has been annotated based on similarity to others, and itself deposited in the database, it can also become the basis for future annotations. This leads to the *transitive annotation problem* because there may be several such annotation transfers by sequence similarity between a particular database record and actual wet lab experimental information. Therefore, one must always regard the biological annotations in major sequence databases with a considerable degree of skepticism, unless they can be verified by reference to published papers describing high-quality experimental data, or at least by reference to a human-curated sequence database.

FASTA Format

In bioinformatics, FASTA format is a text-based format for representing either nucleotide sequences or peptide sequences, in which base pairs or amino acids are represented using single-letter codes. The format also allows for sequence names and comments to precede the sequences.

The simplicity of FASTA format makes it easy to manipulate and parse sequences using text-processing tools and scripting languages like Python, Ruby, and Perl.

Format

The FASTA format may be used to represent either single sequences or many sequences in a single file. A series of single sequences, concatenated, constitute a multisequence file. The best source for a description of the FASTA/Pearson format is the documentation of the FASTA suite of programs. It can be downloaded with any free distribution of FASTA and consult it yourself.

A sequence in FASTA format is represented as a series of lines, which should be no longer than 120 characters and usually do not exceed 80 characters. This probably was because to allow for preallocation of fixed line sizes in software: at the time most users relied on DEC VT (or compatible) terminals which could display 80 or 132 characters per line. Most people preferred the bigger font in 80-character modes and so it became the recommended fashion to use 80 characters or less (often 70) in FASTA lines.

The first line in a FASTA file starts either with a ">" (greater than) symbol or a ";" (semicolon) and was taken as a comment. Subsequent lines starting with a semicolon would be ignored by software. Since the only comment used was the first, it quickly became used to hold a summary description of the sequence, often starting with a unique library accession number, and with time it has become commonplace use to always use ">" for the first line and to not use ";" comments (which would otherwise be ignored).

Following the initial line (used for a unique description of the sequence) is the actual sequence itself in standard one-letter code. Anything other than a valid code would be ignored (including spaces, tabulators, asterisks, etc...). Originally it was also common to end the sequence with an "*" (asterisk) character (in analogy with use in PIR formatted sequences) and, for the same reason, to leave a blank line between the description and the sequence.

A few sample sequences:

;LCBO - Prolactin precursor - Bovine

; a sample sequence in FASTA format

MDSKGSSQKGSRLLLLLVVSNLLLCQGVVSTPVCPNGPGNCQVSLRDLFDRAVMVSHYIHDLSS
EMFNEFDKRYAQGKGFITMALNSCHTSSLPTPEDKEQAQQTHHEVLMSLILGLLRSWNDPLYHL
VTEVRGMKGAPDAILSRAIEIEEENKRLLEGMEMIFGQVIPGAKETEPYPVWSGLPSLQTKDED
ARYSAFYNLLHCLRRDSSKIDTYLKLLNCRIIYNNNC*

>MCHU - Calmodulin - Human, rabbit, bovine, rat, and chicken

ADQLTEEQIAEFKEAFSLFDKDGDGTITTKELGTVMRSLGQNPTEAELQDMINEVDADGNGTID
FPEFLTMMARKMKDTDSEEEIREAFRVFDKDGNGYISAAELRHVMTNLGEKLTDEEVDEMIREA
DIDGDGQVNYEEFVQMMTAK*

>gi|5524211|gb|AAD44166.1| cytochrome b [Elephas maximus maximus]

LCLYTHIGRNIYYGSYLYSETWNTGIMLLLITMATAFMGYVLPWGQMSFWGATVITNLFSAIPYIGTNLV
EWIWGGFSVDKATLNRFFAFHFILPFTMVALAGVHLTFLHETGSNNPLGLTSDSDKIPFHPYYTIKDFLG
LLILILLLLLALLSPDMLGDPDNHMPADPLNTPLHIKPEWYFLFAYAILRSVPNKLGGVLALFLSIVIL
GLMPFLHTSKHRSMMLRPLSQALFWTLTMDLLTLTWIGSQPVEYPYTIIGQMASILYFSIILAFLPIAGX
IENY

A multiple sequence FASTA format would be obtained by concatenating several single sequence FASTA files. This does not imply a contradiction with the format as only the first line in a FASTA file may start with a ";" or ">", hence forcing all subsequent sequences to start with a ">" in order to be taken as different ones (and further forcing the exclusive reservation of ">" for the sequence definition line. Thus, the examples above may as well be taken as a multisequence file if taken together.

In time, common use has led everybody to rely on a simplified FASTA format as the minimum common practice standard as described henceforth:

A sequence in FASTA format begins with a single-line description, followed by lines of sequence data. The description line is distinguished from the sequence data by a greater-than (">") symbol in the first column. The word following the ">" symbol is the identifier of the sequence, and the rest of the line is the description (both are optional). There should be no space between the ">" and the first letter of the identifier. It is recommended that all lines of text be shorter than 80 characters. The sequence ends if another line starting with a ">" appears; this indicates the start of another sequence. A simple example of one sequence in FASTA format:

>gi|5524211|gb|AAD44166.1| cytochrome b [Elephas maximus maximus]

LCLYTHIGRNIYYGSYLYSEIWNTGIMLLLITMATAFMGYVLPWGQMSFWGATVITNLFSAIPYIGTNLV
EWIWGGFSVDKATLNRFFAFHFILPFTMVALAGVHLTFLHETGSNNPLGLTSDSDKIPFHPYYTIKDFLG
LLILILLLLLALLSPDMLGDPDNHMPADPLNTPLHIKPEWYFLFAYAILRSVPNKLGGVLALFLSIVIL
GLMPFLHTSKHRSMMLRPLSQALFWTLTMDLLTLTWIGSQPVEYPYTIIGQMASILYFSIILAFLPIAGX
IENY

Format Converters

FASTA files can be batch converted to or from MultiFASTA format using tools, some of which are available as freeware. Tools are also available for batch conversion from chromatogram formats (ABI/SCF) to FASTA.

Header Line

The header line, which begins with '>', gives a name and/or a unique identifier for the sequence, and often lots of other information too. Many different sequence databases use standardized headers, which helps when automatically extracting information from the header. The header line may contain more than one header, separated by a ^A (Control-A) character (as in (note: *huge* file)). In the original Pearson FASTA format, one or more comments, distinguished by a semi-colon at the beginning of the line, may occur after the header. Most databases and bioinformatics applications do not recognize these comments and follow the NCBI FASTA specification. An example of a multiple sequence FASTA file follows:

>SEQUENCE_1

MTEITAAMVKELRESTGAGMMDCKNALSETNGDFDKAVQLLREKGLGKAAKKADRLAAEG
LVSVKVSDDFTIAAMRPSYLSYEDLDMTFVENEYKALVAELEKENEERRRLKDPNKPEHK
IPQFASRKQLSDAILKEAEEKIKEELKAQGKPEKIWDNIIPGKMNSFIADNSQLDSKLTL
MGQFYVMDDKKTVEQVIAEKEKEFGGKIKIVEFICFEVGEGLEKKTEDFAAEVAAQL
>SEQUENCE_2

SATVSEINSETDFVAKNDQFIALTKDTTAHIQSNSLQSVEELHSSTINGVKFEEYLKSQI
ATIGENLVVRRFATLKAGANGVVNGYIHTNGRVGVVIAAACDSAEVASKSRDLLRQICMH

Sequence Representation

After the header line and comments, one or more lines may follow describing the sequence: each line of a sequence should have fewer than 80 characters.

Sequences may be protein sequences or nucleic acid sequences, and they can contain gaps or alignment characters.

Sequences are expected to be represented in the standard IUB/IUPAC amino acid and nucleic acid codes, with these exceptions: lower-case letters are accepted and are mapped into upper-case; a single hyphen or dash can be used to represent a gap character; and in amino acid sequences, U and * are acceptable letters.

Numerical digits are not allowed but are used in some databases to indicate the position in the sequence.

The nucleic acid codes supported are:

Nucleic Acid Code	Meaning
A	Adenosine
C	Cytosine
G	Guanine
T	Thymidine
U	Uracil
R	G A (puRine)
Y	T C (pYrimidine)
K	G T (Ketone)
M	A C (aMino group)
S	G C (Strong interaction)
W	A T (Weak interaction)
B	G T C (not A) (B comes after A)
D	G A T (not C) (D comes after C)
H	A C T (not G) (H comes after G)
V	G C A (not T, not U) (V comes after U)
N	A G C T (aNy)
X	masked
-	gap of indeterminate length

The codes supported (24 amino acids and 3 special codes) are:

Amino Acid Code	Meaning
A	Alanine
B	Aspartic acid or Asparagine
C	Cysteine
D	Aspartic acid
E	Glutamic acid
F	Phenylalanine
G	Glycine
H	Histidine
I	Isoleucine
K	Lysine
L	Leucine
M	Methionine
N	Asparagine
O	Pyrrolysine
P	Proline
Q	Glutamine
R	Arginine
S	Serine
T	Threonine
U	Selenocysteine
V	Valine
W	Tryptophan
Y	Tyrosine
Z	Glutamic acid or Glutamine
X	any

- • translation stop
- - gap of indeterminate length

Sequence Identifiers

The NCBI defined a standard for the unique identifier used for the sequence (SeqID) in the header line. The formatdb man page has this to say on the subject: "formatdb will automatically parse the SeqID and create indexes, but the database identifiers in the FASTA definition line must follow the conventions of the FASTA Defline Format."

However they do not give a definitive description of the FASTA defline format. An attempt to create such a format is given below.

GenBank *number* | gb | *accession* | *locus*	g	i	|	g	i	-
EMBL Data Library *number* | emb | *accession* | *locus*	g	i	|	g	i	-
DDBJ, DNA Database of Japan *number* | dbj | *accession* | *locus*	g	i	|	g	i	-
NBRF PIR	pir | | *entry*					
Protein Research Foundation	prf | | *name*					
SWISS-PROT	sp | *accession* | *name*					
Brookhaven Protein Data Bank (1)	pdb | *entry* | *chain*					
Brookhaven Protein Data Bank (2) *entry:chain* | PDBID | CHAIN | SEQUENCE						
Patents	pat | country | number					
GenInfo Backbone Id	bbs | number					
General database identifier	gnl | database | identifier					
NCBI Reference Sequence	ref | accession | locus					
Local Sequence identifier	lcl | identifier					

The vertical bars in the above list are not separators in the sense of the Backus-Naur form, but are part of the format.

File Extension

There is no standard file extension for a text file containing FASTA formatted sequences. The table below shows each extension and its respective meaning.

Extension	Meaning	Notes
fasta	generic fasta	Any generic fasta file. Other extensions can be fa, seq, fsa
fna	fasta nucleic acid	For coding regions of a specific genome, use ffn, but otherwise fna is useful for generically specifying nucleic acids.
ffn	FASTA nucleotide coding regions	Contains coding regions for a genome.

| faa | fasta amino acid | Contains amino acids. A multiple protein fasta file can have the more specific extension mpfa. |
| frn | FASTA non-coding RNA | Contains non-coding RNA regions for a genome, in DNA alphabet eg. tRNA, rRNA |

Distributed Computing

SIMAP

Similarity Matrix of Proteins, or SIMAP, is a database of protein similarities created using distributed computing, which is freely accessible for scientific purposes. SIMAP uses the FASTA algorithm to precalculate protein similarity, while another application uses hidden Markov models to search for Protein domains.

SIMAP is a joint project of the Technical University of Munich and the Helmholtz Zentrum Munchen.

The project usually gets new work units at the beginning of each month. More recently, (2010), inclusion of environmental sequences into the database has required longer periods of activity, several months of continuous work for example. Typically, these updates occur twice each year.

In the fourth quarter of 2010, the project relocated to the University of Vienna. Part of this exercise involved the creation of a project specific URL requiring existing users to detach/reattach to the project.

Computing Platform

SIMAP uses the Berkeley Open Infrastructure for Network Computing (BOINC) distributed computing platform.

Application performance notes:

- Work unit CPU times can vary widely, ranging between 15 minutes and 3 hours.
- Work units are around 600 kB to 1.35 MB each, averaging around 1.20 MB.
- SIMAP provides client software optimized for SSE enabled processors. For older processors non SSE applications are provided but require manual installation steps to be taken. Operating Systems supported by SIMAP are Linux, Windows, Mac OS and other UNIX platforms.

- Since the database has been completed, the work available consists of database updates, and may be intermittant.
- UniProt the universal protein database, a central repository of protein data (Swiss-Prot & TrEMBL & PIR).

UniProt is the *Universal Protein* resource, a central repository of protein data created by combining the Swiss-Prot, TrEMBL and PIR-PSD databases. UniProt is based on protein sequences, many of which are derived from genome sequencing projects. It contains a large amount of information about the biological function of proteins derived from the research literature.

The UniProt Consortium

The UniProt Consortium comprises the European Bioinformatics Institute (EBI), the Swiss Institute of Bioinformatics (SIB), and the Protein Information Resource (PIR). EBI, located at the Wellcome Trust Genome Campus in Hinxton, UK, hosts a large resource of bioinformatics databases and services.

SIB, located in Geneva, Switzerland, maintains the ExPASy (Expert Protein Analysis System) servers that are a central resource for proteomics tools and databases. PIR, hosted by the National Biomedical Research Foundation (NBRF) at the Georgetown University Medical Centre in Washington, DC, USA, is heir to the oldest protein sequence database, Margaret Dayhoff's Atlas of Protein Sequence and Structure, first published in 1965. In 2002, EBI, SIB, and PIR joined forces as the UniProt Consortium.

The roots of UniProt Databases

Each consortium member is heavily involved in protein database maintenance and annotation. Until recently, EBI and SIB together produced the Swiss-Prot and TrEMBL databases, while PIR produced the Protein Sequence Database (PIR-PSD). These databases coexisted with differing protein sequence coverage and annotation priorities.

Swiss-Prot was created in 1986 by Amos Bairoch during his PhD and developed by the Swiss Institute of Bioinformatics and the European Bioinformatics Institute.

Swiss-Prot aimed to provide reliable protein sequences associated with a high level of annotation (such as the description of the function of a protein, its domain structure, post-translational modifications, variants, etc.), a minimal level of redundancy and high level of integration with other databases.

Recognizing that sequence data were being generated at a pace exceeding Swiss-Prot's ability to keep up, TrEMBL (Translated EMBL Nucleotide Sequence Data Library) was created to provide automated annotations for those proteins not in Swiss-Prot. Meanwhile, PIR maintained the PIR-PSD and related databases, including iProClass, a database of protein sequences and curated families.

The consortium members pooled their overlapping resources and expertise, and launched UniProt in December 2003.

Organization of UniProt Databases

UniProt provides four core databases:

UniProtKB

UniProt Knowledgebase (UniProtKB) is a protein database curated by experts, consisting of two sections. UniProtKB/Swiss-Prot (containing reviewed, manually annotated entries) and UniProtKB/ TrEMBL (containing unreviewed, automatically annotated entries). In release 2010_09 of 10th August 2010, UniProtKB/Swiss-Prot contained 519,348 entries, and UniProtKB/TrEMBL contained 11,636,205 entries.

UniProtKB/Swiss-Prot

UniProtKB/Swiss-Prot is a high-quality, manually annotated, non-redundant protein sequence database. It combines information extracted from scientific literature and biocurator-evaluated computational analysis. The aim of UniProtKB/Swiss-Prot is to provide all known relevant information about a particular protein. Annotation is regularly reviewed to keep up with current scientific findings. The manual annotation of an entry involves detailed analysis of the protein sequence and of the scientific literature.

Sequences from the same gene and the same species are merged into the same database entry. Differences between sequences are identified, and their cause documented (for example alternative splicing, natural variation, incorrect initiation sites, incorrect exon boundaries, frameshifts, unidentified conflicts). A range of sequence analysis tools is used in the annotation of UniProtKB/Swiss-Prot entries. Computer-predictions are manually evaluated, and relevant results selected for inclusion in the entry. These predictions include post-translational modifications, transmembrane domains and topology, signal peptides, domain identification, and protein family classification.

Relevant publications are identified by searching databases such as PubMed. The full text of each paper is read, and information is extracted and added to the entry. Annotation arising from the scientific literature includes, but is not limited to:

- Protein and gene names
- Function
- Enzyme-specific information such as catalytic activity, cofactors and catalytic residues
- Subcellular location
- Protein-protein interactions
- Pattern of expression
- Locations and roles of significant domains and sites
- Ion-, substrate- and cofactor-binding sites
- Protein variant forms produced by natural genetic variation, RNA editing, alternative splicing, proteolytic processing, and post-translational modification.

Annotated entries undergo quality assurance before inclusion into UniProtKB/Swiss-Prot. When new data becomes available, entries are updated.

UniProtKB/TrEMBL

UniProtKB/TrEMBL contains high-quality computationally analysed records, which are enriched with automatic annotation. It was introduced in response to increased dataflow resulting from genome projects, as the time- and labour-consuming manual annotation process of UniProtKB/Swiss-Prot could not be broadened to include all available protein sequences. The translations of annotated coding sequences in the EMBL-Bank/GenBank/DDBJ nucleotide sequence database are automatically processed and entered in UniProtKB/TrEMBL. UniProtKB/TrEMBL also contains sequences from PDB, and from gene prediction, including Ensembl, RefSeq and CCDS.

UniParc

UniProt Archive (UniParc) is a comprehensive and non-redundant database, which contains all the protein sequences from the main, publicly available protein sequence databases. Proteins may exist in several different source databases, and in multiple copies in the same database. In order to avoid redundancy, UniParc stores each unique sequence only once. Identical sequences are merged, regardless of whether they are from the same or different species.

Each sequence is given a stable and unique identifier (UPI), making it possible to identify the same protein from different source databases. UniParc contains only protein sequences, with no annotation. Database cross-references in UniParc entries allow further information about the protein to be retrieved from the source databases. When sequences in the source databases change, these changes are tracked by UniParc and history of all changes is archived.

Source Databases

Currently UniParc contains protein sequences from the following publicly available databases:

- EMBL-Bank/DDBJ/GenBank nucleotide sequence databases
- Ensembl
- European Patent Office (EPO)
- FlyBase
- H-Invitational Database (H-Inv)
- International Protein Index (IPI)
- Japan Patent Office (JPO)
- PIR-PSD
- Protein Data Bank (PDB)
- Protein Research Foundation (PRF)
- RefSeq
- Saccharomyces Genome database (SGD)
- TAIR Arabidopsis thaliana Information Resource
- TROME
- USA Patent Office (USPTO)
- UniProtKB/Swiss-Prot, UniProtKB/Swiss-Prot protein isoforms, UniProtKB/TrEMBL
- Vertebrate Genome Annotation database (VEGA)
- Worm Base.

UniRef

The UniProt Reference Clusters (UniRef) consist of three databases of clustered sets of protein sequences from UniProtKB and selected UniParc records. The UniRef100 database combines identical sequences and sequence fragments (from any organism) into a single UniRef entry. The sequence of a representative protein, the accession numbers of all the merged entries and links to the corresponding UniProtKB and UniParc records are displayed. UniRef100 sequences are clustered using the CD-HIT algorithm to build UniRef90 and UniRef50. Each cluster is composed of sequences that have at least 90% or 50% sequence identity, respectively, to the longest sequence. Clustering sequences significantly reduces database size, enabling faster sequence searches.

UniMes

The UniProt Metagenomic and Environmental Sequences (UniMES) database is a repository specifically developed for metagenomic and environmental data. The predicted proteins from this dataset are combined with automatic classification by InterPro to enhance the original information with further analysis.

UniProtKB contains protein sequences from known species, data arising from metagenomics studies is from environmental (i.e. uncultured) samples and as such the species may not be known/ identified. UniMES was developed for this data. Data from UniMES is not included in UniProtKB or UniRef, but is included in UniParc. UniMES includes data from the Global Ocean Sampling Expedition (GOS).

Funding for UniProt

UniProt is funded by grants from the National Human Genome Research Institute, the National Institutes of Health (NIH), the European Commission, the Swiss Federal Government through the Federal Office of Education and Science, NCI-caBIG, and the Department of Defence.

Data Mining and Visualisation

Data mining, *the extraction of hidden predictive information from large databases,* is a powerful new technology with great potential to help companies focus on the most important information in their data warehouses.

Data mining tools predict future trends and Behaviours, allowing businesses to make proactive, knowledge-driven decisions. The automated, prospective analyses offered by data mining move beyond the analyses of past events provided by retrospective tools typical of decision support systems.

Data mining tools can answer business questions that traditionally were too time consuming to resolve. They scour databases for hidden patterns, finding predictive information that experts may miss because it lies outside their expectations.

Most companies already collect and refine massive quantities of data. Data mining techniques can be implemented rapidly on existing software and hardware platforms to enhance the value of existing information resources, and can be integrated with new products and systems as they are brought on-line.

When implemented on high performance client/server or parallel processing computers, data mining tools can analyse massive databases to deliver answers to questions such as, "Which clients are most likely to respond to my next promotional mailing, and why?"

This white paper provides an introduction to the basic technologies of data mining. Examples of profitable applications illustrate its relevance to today's business environment as well as a basic description of how data warehouse architectures can evolve to deliver the value of data mining to end users.

The Foundations of Data Mining

Data mining techniques are the result of a long process of research and product development. This evolution began when business data was first stored on computers, continued with improvements in data access, and more recently, generated technologies that allow users to navigate through their data in real time. Data mining takes this evolutionary process beyond retrospective data access and navigation to prospective and proactive information delivery. Data mining is ready for application in the business community because it is supported by three technologies that are now sufficiently mature:

- Massive data collection
- Powerful multiprocessor computers
- Data mining algorithms.

Commercial databases are growing at unprecedented rates. A recent META Group survey of data warehouse projects found that 19% of respondents are beyond the 50 gigabyte level, while 59% expect to be there by second quarter of 1996.1 In some industries, such as retail, these numbers can be much larger.

The accompanying need for improved computational engines can now be met in a cost-effective manner with parallel multiprocessor computer technology. Data mining algorithms embody techniques that have existed for at least 10 years, but have only recently been implemented as mature, reliable, understandable tools that consistently outperform older statistical methods.

In the evolution from business data to business information, each new step has built upon the previous one. For example, dynamic data access is critical for drill-through in data navigation applications, and the ability to store large databases is critical to data mining.

The core components of data mining technology have been under development for decades, in research areas such as statistics, artificial intelligence, and machine learning. Today, the maturity of these techniques, coupled with high-performance relational database engines and broad data integration efforts, make these technologies practical for current data warehouse environments.

The Scope of Data Mining

Data mining derives its name from the similarities between searching for valuable business information in a large database — for example, finding linked products in gigabytes of store scanner data — and mining a mountain for a vein of valuable ore. Both processes require either sifting through an immense amount of material, or intelligently probing it to find exactly where the value resides. Given databases of sufficient size and quality, data mining technology can generate new business opportunities by providing these capabilities:

- Automated prediction of trends and Behaviours. Data mining automates the process of finding predictive information in large databases. Questions that traditionally required extensive hands-on analysis can now be answered directly from the data — quickly. A typical example of a predictive problem is targeted marketing. Data mining uses data on past promotional mailings to identify the targets most likely to maximize return on investment in future mailings. Other predictive problems include forecasting bankruptcy and other forms of default, and identifying segments of a population likely to respond similarly to given events.

- Automated discovery of previously unknown patterns. Data mining tools sweep through databases and identify previously hidden patterns in one step. An example of pattern discovery is the analysis of retail sales data to identify seemingly unrelated products that are often purchased together. Other pattern discovery problems include detecting fraudulent credit card transactions and identifying anomalous data that could represent data entry keying errors.

Data mining techniques can yield the benefits of automation on existing software and hardware platforms, and can be implemented on new systems as existing platforms are upgraded and new products developed. When data mining tools are implemented on high performance parallel processing systems, they can analyse massive databases in minutes. Faster processing means that users can automatically experiment with more models to understand complex data. High speed makes it practical for users to analyse huge quantities of data. Larger databases, in turn, yield improved predictions.

Databases can be larger in both depth and breadth:

- More columns. Analysts must often limit the number of variables they examine when doing hands-on analysis due to time constraints. Yet variables that are discarded because they seem unimportant may carry information about unknown patterns. High performance data mining allows users to explore the full depth of a database, without preselecting a subset of variables.
- More rows. Larger samples yield lower estimation errors and variance, and allow users to make inferences about small but important segments of a population.

A recent Gartner Group Advanced Technology Research Note listed data mining and artificial intelligence at the top of the five key technology areas that "will clearly have a major impact across a wide range of industries within the next 3 to 5 years."2 Gartner also listed parallel architectures and data mining as two of the top 10 new technologies in which companies will invest during the next 5 years. According to a recent Gartner HPC Research Note, "With the rapid advance in data capture, transmission and storage, large-systems users will increasingly need to implement new and innovative ways to mine the after-market value of their vast stores of detail data, employing MPP [massively parallel processing] systems to create new sources of business advantage (0.9 probability)."

The most commonly used techniques in data mining are:

- Artificial neural networks: Non-linear predictive models that learn through training and resemble biological neural networks in structure.

- Decision trees: Tree-shaped structures that represent sets of decisions. These decisions generate rules for the classification of a dataset. Specific decision tree methods include Classification and Regression Trees (CART) and Chi Square Automatic Interaction Detection (CHAID).

- Genetic algorithms: Optimization techniques that use processes such as genetic combination, mutation, and natural selection in a design based on the concepts of evolution.

- Nearest neighbour method: A technique that classifies each record in a dataset based on a combination of the classes of the k record(s) most similar to it in a historical dataset (where k ^{3} 1). Sometimes called the k-nearest neighbour technique.

- Rule induction: The extraction of useful if-then rules from data based on statistical significance.

Many of these technologies have been in use for more than a decade in specialized analysis tools that work with relatively small volumes of data. These capabilities are now evolving to integrate directly with industry-standard data warehouse and OLAP platforms. The appendix to this white paper provides a glossary of data mining terms.

How Data Mining Works

How exactly is data mining able to tell you important things that you didn't know or what is going to happen next? The technique that is used to perform these feats in data mining is called modelling. Modelling is simply the act of building a model in one situation where you know the answer and then applying it to another situation that you don't. For instance, if you were looking for a sunken Spanish galleon on the high seas the first thing you might do is to research the times when Spanish treasure had been found by others in the past. You might note that these ships often tend to be found off the coast of Bermuda and that there are certain characteristics to the ocean currents, and certain routes that have likely been taken by the ship's captains in that era. You note these similarities and build a model that includes the characteristics that are common to the locations of these sunken treasures.

With these models in hand you sail off looking for treasure where your model indicates it most likely might be given a similar situation in the past. Hopefully, if you've got a good model, you find your treasure.

This act of model building is thus something that people have been doing for a long time, certainly before the advent of computers or data mining technology. What happens on computers, however, is not much different than the way people build models. Computers are loaded up with lots of information about a variety of situations where an answer is known and then the data mining software on the computer must run through that data and distill the characteristics of the data that should go into the model.

Once the model is built it can then be used in similar situations where you don't know the answer. For example, say that you are the director of marketing for a telecommunications company and you'd like to acquire some new long distance phone customers.

You could just randomly go out and mail coupons to the general population-just as you could randomly sail the seas looking for sunken treasure. In neither case would you achieve the results you desired and of course you have the opportunity to do much better than random- you could use your business experience stored in your database to build a model.

As the marketing director you have access to a lot of information about all of your customers: their age, sex, credit history and long distance calling usage. The good news is that you also have a lot of information about your prospective customers: their age, sex, credit history etc. Your problem is that you don't know the long distance calling usage of these prospects (since they are most likely now customers of your competition). You'd like to concentrate on those prospects who have large amounts of long distance usage. You can accomplish this by building a model.

The goal in prospecting is to make some calculated guesses about the information in the lower right hand quadrant based on the model that we build going from Customer General Information to Customer Proprietary Information. For instance, a simple model for a telecommunications company might be:

98% of my customers who make more than $60,000/year spend more than $80/month on long distance.

This model could then be applied to the prospect data to try to tell something about the proprietary information that this telecommunications company does not currently have access to. With this model in hand new customers can be selectively targeted.

Test marketing is an excellent source of data for this kind of modelling. Mining the results of a test market representing a broad but relatively small sample of prospects can provide a foundation for identifying good prospects in the overall market.

If someone told you that he had a model that could predict customer usage how would you know if he really had a good model? The first thing you might try would be to ask him to apply his model to your customer base- where you already knew the answer. With data mining, the best way to accomplish this is by setting aside some of your data in a vault to isolate it from the mining process. Once the mining is complete, the results can be tested against the data held in the vault to confirm the model's validity. If the model works, its observations should hold for the vaulted data.

An Architecture for Data Mining

To best apply these advanced techniques, they must be fully integrated with a data warehouse as well as flexible interactive business analysis tools. Many data mining tools currently operate outside of the warehouse, requiring extra steps for extracting, importing, and analysing the data. Furthermore, when new insights require operational implementation, integration with the warehouse simplifies the application of results from data mining.

The resulting analytic data warehouse can be applied to improve business processes throughout the organization, in areas such as promotional campaign management, fraud detection, new product rollout, and so on.

The ideal starting point is a data warehouse containing a combination of internal data tracking all customer contact coupled with external market data about competitor activity. Background information on potential customers also provides an excellent basis for prospecting. This warehouse can be implemented in a variety of relational database systems: Sybase, Oracle, Redbrick, and so on, and should be optimized for flexible and fast data access.

An OLAP (On-Line Analytical Processing) server enables a more sophisticated end-user business model to be applied when navigating the data warehouse. The multidimensional structures allow the user to analyse the data as they want to view their business – summarizing by product line, region, and other key perspectives of their business. The Data Mining Server must be integrated with the data warehouse and the OLAP server to embed ROI-focused business analysis directly into this infrastructure.

An advanced, process-centric metadata template defines the data mining objectives for specific business issues like campaign management, prospecting, and promotion optimization. Integration with the data warehouse enables operational decisions to be directly implemented and tracked. As the warehouse grows with new decisions and results, the organization can continually mine the best practices and apply them to future decisions.

This design represents a fundamental shift from conventional decision support systems. Rather than simply delivering data to the end user through query and reporting software, the Advanced Analysis Server applies users' business models directly to the warehouse and returns a proactive analysis of the most relevant information. These results enhance the metadata in the OLAP Server by providing a dynamic metadata layer that represents a distilled view of the data. Reporting, visualization, and other analysis tools can then be applied to plan future actions and confirm the impact of those plans.

Profitable Applications

A wide range of companies have deployed successful applications of data mining. While early adopters of this technology have tended to be in information-intensive industries such as financial services and direct mail marketing, the technology is applicable to any company looking to leverage a large data warehouse to better manage their customer relationships. Two critical factors for success with data mining are: a large, well-integrated data warehouse and a well-defined understanding of the business process within which data mining is to be applied (such as customer prospecting, retention, campaign management, and so on).

Some successful application areas include:

- A pharmaceutical company can analyse its recent sales force activity and their results to improve targeting of high-value physicians and determine which marketing activities will have the greatest impact in the next few months. The data needs to include competitor market activity as well as information about the local health care systems. The results can be distributed to the sales force via a wide-area network that enables the representatives to review the recommendations from the perspective of the key attributes in the decision process. The ongoing, dynamic analysis of the data warehouse allows best practices from throughout the organization to be applied in specific sales situations.

- A credit card company can leverage its vast warehouse of customer transaction data to identify customers most likely to be interested in a new credit product. Using a small test mailing, the attributes of customers with an affinity for the product can be identified. Recent projects have indicated more than a 20-fold decrease in costs for targeted mailing campaigns over conventional approaches.

- A diversified transportation company with a large direct sales force can apply data mining to identify the best prospects for its services. Using data mining to analyse its own customer experience, this company can build a unique segmentation identifying the attributes of high-value prospects. Applying this segmentation to a general business database such as those provided by Dun & Bradstreet can yield a prioritized list of prospects by region.

- A large consumer package goods company can apply data mining to improve its sales process to retailers. Data from consumer panels, shipments, and competitor activity can be applied to understand the reasons for brand and store switching. Through this analysis, the manufacturer can select promotional strategies that best reach their target customer segments.

Each of these examples have a clear common ground. They leverage the knowledge about customers implicit in a data warehouse to reduce costs and improve the value of customer relationships. These organizations can now focus their efforts on the most important (profitable) customers and prospects, and design targeted marketing strategies to best reach them.

Conclusion

Comprehensive data warehouses that integrate operational data with customer, supplier, and market information have resulted in an explosion of information. Competition requires timely and sophisticated analysis on an integrated view of the data.

However, there is a growing gap between more powerful storage and retrieval systems and the users' ability to effectively analyse and act on the information they contain. Both relational and OLAP technologies have tremendous capabilities for navigating massive data warehouses, but brute force navigation of data is not enough.

A new technological leap is needed to structure and prioritize information for specific end-user problems. The data mining tools can make this leap. Quantifiable business benefits have been proven through the integration of data mining with current information systems, and new products are on the horizon that will bring this integration to an even wider audience of users.

Glossary of Data Mining Terms

analytical model	A structure and process for analysing a dataset. For example, a decision tree is a model for the classification of a dataset.
anomalous data	Data that result from errors (for example, data entry keying errors) or that represent unusual events. Anomalous data should be examined carefully because it may carry important information.
artificial neural networks	Non-linear predictive models that learn through training and resemble biological neural networks in structure.
CART	Classification and Regression Trees. A decision tree technique used for classification of a dataset. Provides a set of rules that you can apply to a new (unclassified) dataset to predict which records will have a given outcome. Segments a dataset by creating 2-

way splits. Requires less data preparation than CHAID.

CHAID

Chi Square Automatic Interaction Detection. A decision tree technique used for classification of a dataset. Provides a set of rules that you can apply to a new (unclassified) dataset to predict which records will have a given outcome. Segments a dataset by using chi square tests to create multi-way splits. Preceded, and requires more data preparation than, CART.

classification

The process of dividing a dataset into mutually exclusive groups such that the members of each group are as "close" as possible to one another, and different groups are as "far" as possible from one another, where distance is measured with respect to specific variable(s) you are trying to predict. For example, a typical classification problem is to divide a database of companies into groups that are as homogeneous as possible with respect to a creditworthiness variable with values "Good" and "Bad."

clustering

The process of dividing a dataset into mutually exclusive groups such that the members of each group are as "close" as possible to one another, and different groups are as "far" as possible from one another, where distance is measured with respect to all available variables.

data cleansing

The process of ensuring that all values in a dataset are consistent and correctly recorded.

data mining

The extraction of hidden predictive information from large databases.

data navigation

The process of viewing different dimensions, slices, and levels of detail of a multidimensional database.

data visualization

The visual interpretation of complex relationships in multidimensional data.

data warehouse

A system for storing and delivering massive quantities of data.

decision tree	A tree-shaped structure that represents a set of decisions. These decisions generate rules for the classification of a dataset.
dimension	In a flat or relational database, each field in a record represents a dimension. In a multidimensional database, a dimension is a set of similar entities; for example, a multidimensional sales database might include the dimensions Product, Time, and City.
exploratory data analysis	The use of graphical and descriptive statistical techniques to learn about the structure of a dataset.
genetic algorithms	Optimization techniques that use processes such as genetic combination, mutation, and natural selection in a design based on the concepts of natural evolution.
linear model	An analytical model that assumes linear relationships in the coefficients of the variables being studied.
linear regression	A statistical technique used to find the best-fitting linear relationship between a target (dependent) variable and its predictors (independent variables).
logistic regression	A linear regression that predicts the proportions of a categorical target variable, such as type of customer, in a population.
multidimensional database	A database designed for on-line analytical processing. Structured as a multidimensional hypercube with one axis per dimension.
multiprocessor computer	A computer that includes multiple processors connected by a network.
nearest neighbour	A technique that classifies each record in a dataset based on a combination of the classes of the k record(s) most similar to it in a historical dataset (where k ³ 1). Sometimes called a k-nearest neighbour technique.
non-linear model	An analytical model that does not assume linear relationships in the coefficients of the variables being studied.

OLAP	On-line analytical processing. Refers to array-oriented database applications that allow users to view, navigate through, manipulate, and analyse multidimensional databases.
outlier	A data item whose value falls outside the bounds enclosing most of the other corresponding values in the sample. May indicate anomalous data. Should be examined carefully; may carry important information.
parallel processing	The coordinated use of multiple processors to perform computational tasks. Parallel processing can occur on a multiprocessor computer or on a network of workstations or PCs.
predictive model	A structure and process for predicting the values of specified variables in a dataset.
prospective data analysis	Data analysis that predicts future trends, Behaviours, or events based on historical data.
RAID	Redundant Array of Inexpensive Disks. A technology for the efficient parallel storage of data for high-performance computer systems.
retrospective data analysis	Data analysis that provides insights into trends, Behaviours, or events that have already occurred.
rule induction	The extraction of useful if-then rules from data based on statistical significance.
SMP	Symmetric multiprocessor. A type of multiprocessor computer in which memory is shared among the processors.
terabyte	One trillion bytes.
time series analysis	The analysis of a sequence of measurements made at specified time intervals. Time is usually the dominating dimension of the data.

Twenty years ago, only experts could create computer images of a protein structure at atomic detail, a large phylogenetic tree, or a complex biochemical pathway.

Today, software tools for creating these images are widely available and widely used. Of the different visualization areas in biology, molecular graphics is perhaps the most mature, and as a result, molecular graphic images are widely used in textbooks, presentations and popular media.

Other fields, such as genome visualization, are much younger; however, even here, molecular biologists have a rich toolbox of visualization software at their disposal, many of these tools amenable to use by non-experts.

A main reason for the increased accessibility and use of visualization software has been the advances in computer hardware and network access. Many visualization tasks that previously required expensive and specialized hardware can now be easily managed with a standard personal computer. However, an equally important factor has been the development of a wide range of methods and tools specialized in visualizing specific kinds of biological data.

In this Supplement, we discuss over 200 tools selected from the much greater number now available. This diversity of tools can be confusing, but it is probably unavoidable, given the diverse nature of the biosciences. In fact, in many cases, biologists still find that their exact requirements are not met by current tools and often have to create custom solutions. This has helped spur a growing trend to allow reuse of visualization software, either by means of open source software libraries or by means of architectures specifically designed to allow extensions.

Integration is Improving

In the past, visualization tools were typically stand-alone programs designed to view data from a single experiment. In contrast, many of today's tools are integrated with remote databases and provide visualizations that integrate data from multiple sources.

For instance, Jalview—a popular tool for editing multiple sequence alignments—can connect to multiple data sources and displays not only alignments but also a wide variety of sequence feature information.

In addition, tools are increasingly being designed to interoperate directly with other visualization and analysis tools. Such interoperation can enable, for example, simultaneous interactive visualization of a multiple sequence alignment with corresponding three-dimensional structures—or of a network with corresponding heat maps, profile plots or phylogenetic trees and dendrograms.

Finally, many of today's visualization tools can be either directly embedded into, or launched from, web pages; and such tools are being used to construct integrated web applications for data mining and browsing, often using multiple visualization tools.

For example, the UCSC Genome Browser shows genomic sequences assembled from many laboratories and provides access to a diverse range of related data, including multiple sequence alignments among sequences from similar organisms, three-dimensional structures and *in situ* hybridization images.

The improved integration in visualization tools has been helped greatly by a trend toward increased consolidation of experimental data. An exemplary case of this trend is macromolecular three-dimensional structure: almost all experimentally determined structures are consolidated in a single resource (wwPDB9).

Unfortunately, such consolidation is still the exception: it is more typical in biology to have equivalent data distributed over many resources. In the case of image data from high-throughput experiments, most of these data are never made publicly available, even though this would clearly be of value. Some preliminary steps are being made, but a truly consolidated resource for image data is likely to remain a distant goal owing to difficulties with defining standards for organizing and categorizing these data and to data set sizes that are prohibitively large for network-based transfer.

User-interface Challenges

Although visualization methods and tools have greatly improved, there has also been an exponential increase in the size and complexity of data sets studied in biology. A common challenge faced by many biologists is how to benefit from this data deluge without being overwhelmed by it. Visualization is clearly part of the solution; however, the sheer number and diversity of tools available can make the problem worse. Below we discuss several recent advances toward addressing these issues.

Usability. Very often, biologists fail to fully benefit from visualization methods because software tools are too difficult to learn. Making software that is easy to use often requires considerable work.

Fortunately, there have been many advances in understanding principles of software usability.

These principles are increasingly being adopted by developers of visualization tools for biologists. Judging from progress over the past decade, we expect the usability standard to continue to improve. Unfortunately, improvements may be slow, because work on usability is usually less rewarded in science than is research on new methods.

Visual analytics. In the process of understanding and interpreting biological data, tools ideally would provide visualization for tasks that require human judgment, and other tasks would be automated where possible.

But, finding a productive balance between automation and visualization is a challenge and is one of the goals of visual analytics methods, which involve studying the role of visualization in the whole process of analysing and understanding data.

Recently, these methods have begun to be applied to biological visualization tools, and, if successful, these developments will improve the ability of tools to provide meaningful biological insights and to meet user requirements.

Multiscale representation and navigation. Biological data visualization often deals with a broad range of scales—for example, images may range from the atomic scale to the cellular level and genomic browsers provide information from whole chromosomes down to an individual nucleotide position.

To be useful, the graphical representations used need to adjust, ideally displaying the level of detail appropriate to a particular scale. For example, in showing the threedimensional structure of a protein, ribbon representation is often used to hide all atoms except those involved in ligand interactions; as a user zooms out to see higher-order protein complexes, ribbon representation is too detailed and is replaced by an overall surface.

Although the basic ideas are not new, the details of how to realize multiscale navigation vary greatly with the data type. This is the subject of ongoing research, particularly in visualizing genomic data, pathways and networks and joint visualization of image data sets acquired at different resolution, requiring multimodal image registration. Innovative representations.

In all areas of biology, new visual metaphors and graphical representations are being developed to convey information and to facilitate navigation. Innovation of representations is often inspired by the need to visualize new types of data or to support new analysis tasks.

Examples include the need to display expression profile data together with pathway data (Gehlenborg et al.4) or the need to make genome assembly structures easier to see. In some cases, the innovations are brought in from outside of biology; for instance, partial order graphs are representations taken from discrete mathematics that are now being used to create concise summaries of multiple alignment information and to visualize alternative gene splicing.

Standardized representations. Because visualization methods are still rapidly evolving, part of the difficulty faced by end users today arises from a lack of standards in representations.

Although there is an obvious strength in diversity, and indeed a need for continued innovation in graphical representation, in many cases usability would be enhanced by the adoption of some standards in representation. In systems biology, there has recently been a significant community-driven proposal toward developing a more unified standard for graphical notation of biochemical networks, and we anticipate similar proposals in other areas.

Display hardware. To help display and use complex biological data sets, large display devices and tiled arrays with improved resolution are likely to be of significant benefit. As these devices become more affordable, they are likely to see more use.

Adding a third dimension. The use of threedimensional visualization is being explored for networks, phylogenetic trees and genomics data. Although the third dimension adds complexity to the user interface, three-dimensional visualization may be necessary for some very complex data sets. Visualization in three dimensions is helped greatly by hardware stereo, which is now becoming easily affordable.

Augmented computer interaction. For challenging data sets, we anticipate the increased use of methods that augment or improve the ability to interact with visual data. For example, tangible devices that give touch feedback are becoming more affordable and are promising for three-dimensional structure visualization. Preliminary studies on augmenting visualization with auditory techniques ('sonification') have also been done, using molecular three-dimensional structure and sequence information.

Computational Challenges

Today, many visualization tasks are easily accomplished using a standard personal computer. However, in almost all areas of biology, visualization of cutting-edge data sets remains a challenge. For instance, a modern high-throughput image data set may consist of thousands of videos or hundreds of channels (each channel typically corresponding to one gene product)—and may be up to tens of terabytes in size. To interactively visualize these data, personal computers are often inadequate.

This situation is inspiring further innovation in software— especially in methods for dimension reduction and classification, which underlie visualization tools in many areas of biology. For example, the recently developed MCL clustering algorithm— which enables fast network clustering—has been implemented in a range of visualization tools, particularly in systems biology.

Although these advances will undoubtedly improve on today's limitations, our ability to collect data will also continue to improve, and it is certain to continually challenge our visualization capabilities.

Future Visualization

Ultimately, the goal of visualizing biological data is to provide biologists with an integrated framework they can use to gain insight into the processes in organelles, cells, organs and even whole organisms. Fulfilling this ambitious goal requires substantial further development in visualization methods, especially better integration of different tool types.

Several efforts to build such integrated visualization frameworks have begun—for example, using the framework of genomic coordinates to integrate increasingly diverse data. Other frameworks based on commonly used systems biology data types are being developed.

And projects from the structural biology and microscopy communities aim to integrate biological data on the basis of a cellular coordinate framework by synthesizing multiscale data, including data from cellular tomograms, cryo-electron microscopy, and atomic-detail three-dimensional structures, as well as inventories of expressed proteins, estimations of organelle shapes and distributions, and protein localizations and gradients.

Probably no single framework will suit all biologists; however, the goals of these different efforts may eventually produce a standardized visualization environment that allows seamless integration of biological data.

Creating such integrated visualization frameworks will require a collective effort, and several initiatives toward collaborative, community-based editing of biological image data have already begun. But all these efforts are still very much at the pioneering stage, and, to paraphrase Alan Kay, we could say that the revolution in biological data visualization hasn't started yet.

Bibliography

Aldridge, S.: *The Thread of Life: The Story of Genes and Genetic Engineering*, Cambridge University Press, Cambridge, 1996.

Allan, V., B. Backley, L. Felperin, N. James and H. Gee: *Sight and Sound Supplement*, BFI, London, 1996.

Astor, G.: *The "Last" Nazi: The Life and Times of Dr. Joseph Mengele*, Weidenfeld and Nicolson, London, 1985.

Ayala, F. J.: *The Genetic Structure of Populations*, W.H. Freeman & Co., San Francisco, California, 1977.

Bajema, C. J.: *Natural Selection in Human Populations, the Measurement of Ongoing Genetic Evolution in Contemporary Societies*, Wiley, New York, 1971.

Barnaby, W.: *Plague Makers: The Secret World of Biological Warfare*, Vision Paperbacks, London, 1999.

Bast, R.C. Jr.: *Cancer Medicine*, Decker, Hamilton, 2000.

Bauer, M.: *Resistance to New Technology: Nuclear Power, Information Technology and Biotechnology*, Cambridge University Press, Cambridge, England, 1995.

Berg, Paul, and Singer, Maxine: *Dealing with Genes: The Language of Heredity. Mill Valley*, University Science Books, CA, 1992.

Bernard, C.: *An Introduction to the Study of Experimental Medicine*, Dover Publications, New York, 1957.

Berry, R. J.: *Inheritance and Natural History*: Collins, London, 1977.

Bradley, W.G.: *Neurology in Clinical Practice*, Butterworth Heinemann, Boston, 2000.

Branagh, K., S. Lady, and F. Darabont: *Mary Shelley's Frankenstein: The Classic Tale of Terror Reborn*, Newmarket Press, London, 1994.

Brookes, Martin: *Get a Grip on Genetics, Time Life Books*, East Sussex, England, 1998.

Brosnan, J.: *The Primal Scream: A History of Science Fiction Film*, Orbit Books, London, 1991.

Bukatman, S.: *Blade Runner*, BFI, London, 1997.

Campbell, Neil A.; Brad Williamson; Robin J. Heyden: *Biology: Exploring Life*, Pearson Prentice Hall, Boston, Massachusetts, 2006.

Crick, F.: *Life Itself: Its Origin and Nature*, W.W. Norton, New York, 1982.

Curtis, M.: *The Geometry of DNA: A Structural Revision*, Blue Gallery, London, 1996.

Dams, R.D.: *Principles of Neurology*, McGraw Hill, New York, 1997.

Dawkins, R.: *The Selfish Gene*, Oxford University Press, New York, 1976.

Diaz, E.: *Microbial Biodegradation: Genomics and Molecular Biology*, Caister Academic Press, UK, 2008.

Dobzhanshy, T.: *Genetics of the Evolutionary Process*, Columbia University Press, New York, 1970.

Dulbecco, R.: *The Design of Life*, Yale University Press, New Haven, Connecticut, 1987.

Dunbar, Robert E.: *Heredity*, Franklin Watts Publisher, New York, 1978.

Edey, M. A., and Johanson, D. C.: *Blueprints: Solving the Mystery of Evolution*, Little, Brown and Co., Boston, Mass, 1989.

Fisher, R. A.: *The Genetical Theory of Natural Selection*, Clarendon Press, Oxford, 1930.

Fritz, A.: *International Classification of Diseases for Oncology*, World Health Organization, Geneva, 2000.

Gall, Joseph G.: *Landmark Papers in Cell Biology*, Cold Spring Harbor Laboratory Press, Plainview, NY, 2001.

Garza-Valdes, L.A.: *The DNA of God?* Hodder and Stoughton, London, 1998.

George S. Paul: *Beyond Humanity: Cyber Evolution and Future Minds*, Charles River Media, Roackland, 1996.

Gillis, Justin: *Drug Firms, Gene Labs to Map Genetic Code*, The Daily News, Longview, WA, 1999.

Glover, D. M., and Hames, B. D.: *Genes and Embryos*, Oxford University Press, New York, 1989.

Goldman, L.; Ausiello, D. A.: *Cecil Textbook of Medicine*, Saunders, Philadelphia, 2004.

Griffiths A.J.F.: *Introduction to Genetic Analysis*, W.H. Freeman and Company, New York, USA, 2005.

Halacy, D.S., Jr.: *Genetic Revolution, Shaping Life for Tomorrow*, Harper & Row, Publishers, New York, 1974.

Hamerton, J. L.: *Human Cytogenetics*, Academic Press, New York, 1971.

Hanley, R.: *Is Data Human? The Metaphysics of Star Trek*, Boxtree, London, 1998.

Hartl, Daniel L.: *Basic Genetics*, Jones and Bartlett Publishers, Boston, 1991.

Haubrich, W.S.: *Bockus Gastroenterology*, Saunders, Philadelphia, 1995.

Heider, J. and Rabus, R: *Microbial Biodegradation: Genomics and Molecular Biology*, Caister Academic Press, UK, 2008.

Holtz, Robert D.; William, Kovacs D.: *An Introduction to Geotechnical Engineering*, Prentice Hall, UK, 1981.

Jameson, J. L.: *Principles of Molecular Medicine*, Humana Press, Totowa, 1998.

Jonoska, N.: *Self-Assembling DNA Graphs, DNA-Based Computers VIII*, Springer-Verlag, Berlin, 2003.

Kelves, D.: *In the Name of Eugenics: Genetics and the Uses of Human Heredity*. Harmondsworth: Penguin.

Klein, Aaron E.: *Threads of Life: Genetics from Aristotle to DNA*, The Natural History Press, Garden City, New York, 1955.

Klug, William S. and Michael R.: Cummings. *Essentials of Genetics*, Prentice Hall, New Jersey, 1996.

Lakoff, G. and M. Johnson: *Metaphors We Live By*, University of Chicago Press, Chicago, 1980.

Lewin B.: *Genes VII*, Oxford University Press Inc., New York, USA, 2000.

Lewontin, R.C.: *The Doctrine of DNA: Biology as Ideology*, Penguin, Harmondsworth, 1993.

Lyon, Jeff and Gorner, Peter. Altered Fates: *Gene Therapy and the Retooling of Human Life*, W. W. Norton and Company, New York, 1995.

Margulis, L.: *Symbiosis in Cell Evolution*, W.H. Freeman, San Francisco, 1981.

Mayr, E.: *Change of Genetic Environment and Evolution*, Allen and Unwin, London, 1954.

Mayr, Ernst: *The Growth of Biological Thought: Diversity, Evolution, and Inheritance*, Harvard University Press, Cambridge, 2000.

Migloni, G.S.: *Dictionary of Plant Genetics and Molecular Biology*, Hawthorne Press, New York, 1998.

Nelkin, D. and M.S. Lindee: *The DNA Mystique: The Gene as a Cultural Icon*, W.H. Freeman, New York, 1995.

Nottingham, S.F.: *Eat Your Genes: How Genetically Modified Food is Entering Our Diet*, Zed Books, London, 1998.

Rietman, Ed.: *Molecular Engineering of Nanosystems*, Springer, New York, 2001.

Schummer, J.: *Interdisciplinary Issues in Nanoscale Research*, IOS Press, Amsterdam, 2004.

Scriver, C.R.: *The Metabolic and Molecular Basis of Inherited Disease*, McGraw Hill, New York, 2001.

Stebbins, G. L.: *Darwin to DNA, Molecules to Humanity*, W. H. Freeman, San Francisco, 1982.

Sturtevant, Alfred: *History of Genetics*, Harper and Row, New York, 1965.

Stwertka, Eve and Albert: *Genetic Engineering*, Franklin Watts, New York, 1982.

Suzuki, D., and Knudtson, P.: *Genethics: The Clash Between the New Genetics and Human Values*, Harvard University Press, Cambridge, Mass, 1989.

Watson, J. D.: *The Double Helix*, Antheneum, New York, 1968.

Williams, J.G. and R.K. Patient: *Genetic Engineering*, IRL Press, Oxford, England, 1988.

Wilson, E. O., and Lumden, C.: *Genes, Mind, and Culture: The Evolutionary Process*, Harvard University Press, Cambridge, Mass, 1981.

Wilson, E. O.: *Biophilia*, Harvard University Press, Cambridge, Mass, 1985.

Winchester, A. M.: *Heredity, Evolution and Humankind*, West Publishing Co., St. Paul, Minn., 1976.

Winston, R.: *The Future of Genetic Manipulation*, Phoenix, London, 1997.

Wright, L.: *Twins: Genes, Environment and the Mystery of Human Identity*, Weidenfeld & Nicolson, London, 1997.

Zimmerman, E. G.: *Karyology, Systematics, and Chromosomal Evolution in the Rodent Genus, Sigmodon*, Michigan State Univ., UK 1970.

Index

❑❑❑